LIVING ALONE WITH DEMENTIA—ALZHEIMER'S
(How to Keep Your Loved One in Their Home as Long as Possible)

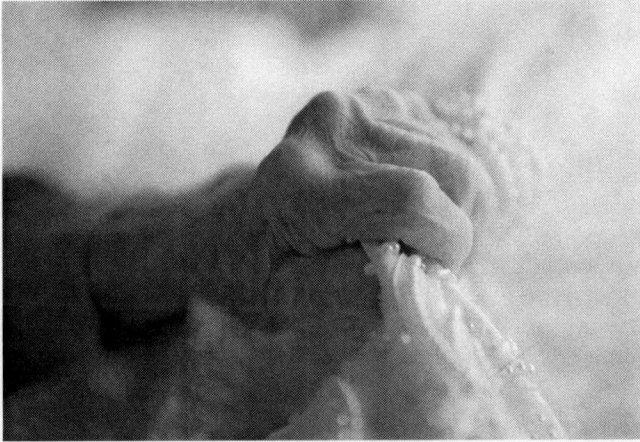

Terry F. Townsend

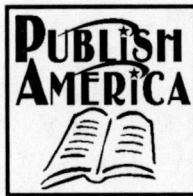

PUBLISH AMERICA

PublishAmerica
Baltimore

First printing

PublishAmerica has allowed this work to remain exactly as the author intended, verbatim, without editorial input.

ISBN: 1-60672-256-5
PUBLISHED BY PUBLISHAMERICA, LLLP
www.publishamerica.com
Baltimore

Printed in the United States of America

In Loving Memory

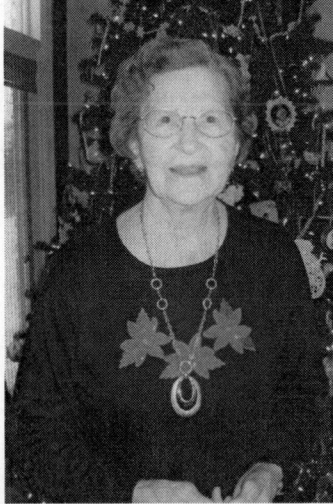

I wish to dedicate this book to my wonderful mother of 86 years of age who has always been there for my two sisters and me. The woman who gave us life and put us on the straight and narrow path by raising us in a Christian home, along with my dad, never wavered. She devoted her life to providing for and doing everything she could to be the best mother possible. We always seemed to be her reason for living, or at least she made us feel that way. My mother and dad were our foundation until my dad passed away in 1974. Mother always worked long, hard hours until she was in her 70's as a retail sales lady for two different department stores. Having spent many long hours on her feet all day on a concrete floor as a retail sales clerk and then coming home to perform her duties as a wife and mother of three, she endured a great deal over the years. My mother never asked anything for herself but was always doing for others. She was always very active in the church, cooking and delivering food, and helping needy members. I think it is accurate to say that toward the end of her life, because of her Alzheimer's, she was no longer mentally the same person we loved all those years. To my sisters and me, however, she will always be the mother that instilled thousands of wonderful memories that we will cherish forever. She finally passed away from heart failure and has now gone on to be with our dad and all her family members who have gone before her but if the good Lord gives out mother awards, she surely received one.

In Loving Memory

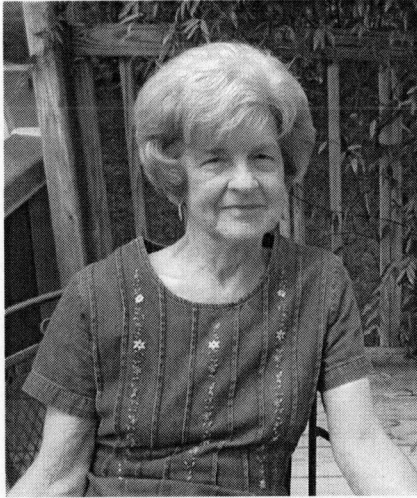

I also wish to dedicate this book to my mother's wonderful sister, Anne Stutts. This wonderful lady was a driving force in assisting my sisters and me with my mother's disease. Her constant phone calls and visits to my mother were invaluable to her and to us. An even greater accomplishment was the tremendous inspiration she was to the entire family by the strength and perseverance and grace she exemplified in her own personal battle with cancer. She never complained about her pain or asked for help in spite of the obvious needs her disease created. She graciously fought a group of cancers for years that had taken over several organs of her body and she finally passed away this past April 2nd. All of us who loved her will always remember her as the little force to be reckoned with by cancer, because she never gave up no matter how tough the disease got.

Preface

I think most of us have a tendency to take many things in our lives for granted such as being fortunate enough to constantly have family living in the home with us. If you live with someone, you have the security of someone to help you if you get sick or develop some disease. This is so very important especially when you put yourself in the shoes of someone who is less fortunate and is forced to live alone. My mother lived alone until she reached the advanced stages of Alzheimer's. Fortunately for her, she had three adult kids who cared enough to constantly help her deal with her condition. It is so very important for those of us who are directly affected by the effects of Alzheimer's or any other type of Dementia on our loved ones, to be ready and able to help them in every way possible. It is my belief that this can best be accomplished by learning all we can about the disease and how to deal with it. If those of us who have gone through this with someone we love or care about can share what we have learned to help others better deal with it in their lives, then we need to make every effort to do it. Over the six years that my mother had this disease, we were forced to learn a great deal about Dementia and how to best handle situations that arose because of it. The more you know about the disease, the better prepared you will be to effectively help someone who has it. Back when my mother was first diagnosed with Alzheimer's, I knew nothing about the disease or the terrible effect it could have on the entire family of someone who had it. It was definitely a learning experience that was constantly on going. Initially, changes became noticeable gradually, and then as time went on, we began to notice changes much more frequently. It became obvious to us that steps needed to be taken periodically to help us keep her in her home as long as we could, which became our goal. I believe we could all agree that in most cases once you remove your loved one from their home, it's almost like their reason for living diminishes much more rapidly. It is my hope that this book will provide valuable information to help anyone with a loved one diagnosed with a mind degenerative disease. It is so very important to find ways to keep them with you mentally as long as absolutely possible and in their own home. I realize that all situations are different to some extent, but each case is similar in many respects as well. It is because of these similarities that we are able to learn things to help others going through the same difficult periods. Now that my mother has left this world, I feel confident in my heart that we did everything possible to assist in making the most difficult years of her life better than they otherwise would have been. I definitely did not want this disease to make her final years with us miserable. I feel that what we learned along the way and implemented as necessary, greatly improved the quality of her life.

Table of Contents

Chapter 1
What Is Dementia 11

Chapter 2
Reduce Your Risk of Alzheimer's/Dementia 15

Chapter 3
Becoming Aware of the First Signs of Dementia 25

Chapter 4
Getting Your Loved One into a Clinical Study 31

Chapter 5
You Begin to Notice Memory Loss 33

Chapter 6
They Begin Repeating Themselves 39

Chapter 7
Losing Things Becomes a Problem 43

Chapter 8
Becoming Disoriented 47

Chapter 9
Forcing Changes on Them, but Doing It Discretely . 51

Chapter 10
Effects on the Family of Someone with Dementia .. 69

Chapter 11
Electronic Devices Can Be Very Helpful 73

Chapter 12
Knowing When It's Time for an In-Home Sitter...... 79

Chapter 13
Going from Home to a Facility in Stages................. 85

Chapter 14
Helpful Resources 91

Chapter 15
Know in Your Heart, You Did Your Best 99

A Little About the Author 103
Bibliography... 105

Chapter 1
WHAT IS DEMENTIA

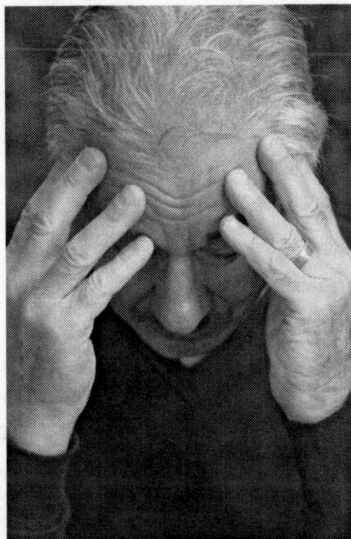

D ementia is a word used for a group of brain disorders that gradually reduce a person's ability to perform daily activities. It is a progressive disorder that takes away a person's memory and their ability to learn and carry out their daily activities. The disease affects the brain in different ways. Some of the symptoms of these diseases include forgetfulness, confusion, trouble organizing or expressing thoughts, and changes in their personality and behavior. Dementia is one of the most common health problems confronting the elderly today. While the cause of Dementia is not yet known, age is the main known risk factor. There are 5.2 million Americans with Alzheimer's, the most common form of Dementia and more than double the number in 1980, and by the year 2050 it is expected that over 16 million Americans will have the disease. Alzheimer's was named after Dr. Alois Alzheimer in 1910. This disease accounts for 50% to 70% of all Dementia cases. It staggers the imagination to think how severe the disease is worldwide. The experts estimate that some 500,000 Americans in their 30's, 40's, & 50's have some form of Dementia, but most of them have Alzheimer's. It mostly affects people who are 65 or older. At age 65 to 74, up to 5% of people have it, while half of those aged 85 and up have the disease.

These statistics enforce the fact that age plays such a major role in this disease. Most all of us have been or will be affected in some way by this terrible disease. We will either get the disease ourselves, someone in our family will, or at least someone we are close to will get the disease in our lifetime. I'm sure that almost everyone knows someone who has the disease or did have it. Many families have had several members who have had this disease, as is the case with my family. Over the years, there have been several members of my mother's side of the family who had Alzheimer's. Strangely enough, most of them have been females with one exception. We first noticed signs of Dementia when my mother was 79 and she passed away at age 86 with advanced stage Alzheimer's.

Dementia creeps into a person's life much like an unsuspected thief in the night. When we attribute a forgotten item or moment, or momentarily forget what we were going to say, as merely getting older, the thief has done his work. In the beginning a person may understand what it means to have been diagnosed with Alzheimer's, but a time soon comes when they no longer realize they have the disease. The disease gradually confiscates the mind without the patient realizing it. A good correlation might be if a painter gradually painted our mind from white to black by way of many varied darkening shades of gray. A person seems to ease into a state of Alzheimer's without even knowing it and in too many cases before their loved ones realize what's happening. At times, it's almost like "now you see them now you don't". This is especially true with loved ones you don't often see. This is just one reason why it is so important to stay in touch with all your family members. If they have close friends, they may notice a problem and contact a family member but there are no guarantees for this.

Of course we all know several famous people who have had it such as Ronald Reagan, Charlton Heston, and Rita Hayworth, just to name a few. Dementia plays no favorites and can strike anyone no matter how much money you have, where you live, the color of your skin or any other group.

Other related forms of Dementia would include Mild Cognitive Impairment (MCI); Vascular Dementia; Mixed Dementia; Dementia with Lewy Bodies; Parkinson's Disease; Frontotemporal Dementia; Creutzfeldt-Jakob Disease (CJD); Normal Pressure Hydrocephalus; Huntington's Disease; and Wernicke-Korsakoff Syndrome.

You can visit the Alzheimer's Association's web site for specific information on any of the above listed forms of Dementia. The link to their web site is http://www.alz.org/alzheimersdiseaserelateddiseases.asp.

Foot Note-Alzheimer's Association web site, What is Alzheimer's?

Chapter 2
REDUCE YOUR RISK OF ALZHEIMER'S/DEMENTIA

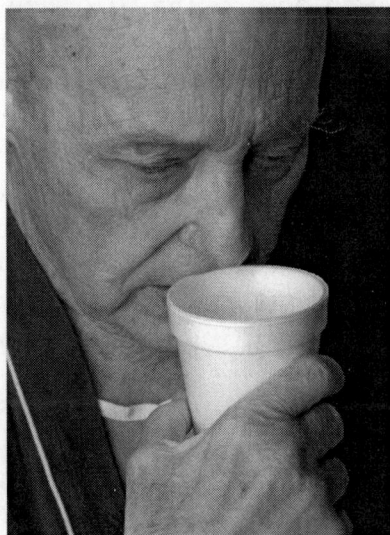

According to Dr. Russell Blaylock, a Physician, Neurosurgeon, author, and health advocate, we should first focus on the importance of exercising our memory to reduce the risk of Alzheimer's, if you don't already have it. Medical scientists cannot explain the acceleration in brain disease cases; however, there are many possible reasons for it. According to Dr. Blaylock, there are common toxins in our environment and even in our kitchen or bathroom that can literally excite our brain cells to death. His good news is that there are some simple steps you can take to reduce your risk by exercising your memory. Here are some steps to follow to help keep your mind alert and active. If you have a loved one who already has this disease, these steps may assist in slowing the degenerative process if they can be coached into performing them. We tried several such steps with my mother and anything you can do to constantly challenge their mind is helpful. Mother used to do a great deal of cooking and much of it from recipes, so we encouraged her in this area because it helped to keep her mind active. She used to love to do crossword puzzles and read the scrolling text that would move across the bottom of the TV screen, but regardless of how small these things seem they were very instrumental in stimulating her mind.

1) Make a conscious effort to be alert. This may sound elementary, but simply being alert to your surroundings exercises your memory. Make every attempt to consistently look around you and notice what is going on. If family members are visiting, pay attention to what they are doing, what they are saying and how they are affecting your life. Try to notice what the weather is doing, what are the birds and squirrels and other critters outside your window doing. Force yourself to notice the traffic on your street or road, and the neighbor's dogs and cats or other livestock. Try to notice when the mailman arrives each day and when the paper gets delivered. Generally make every effort to be aware of what is going on around you in as many different areas as possible.

2) Get as organized as possible. If it's worth memorizing, it's worth taking notes on it. Scientists agree that short-term memory can only hold seven items at one time. Choose your seven and write down notes about others. For example, most people can remember as many as seven items to purchase at the grocery store but more than that should be written down. If you have several tasks that you plan to do in a given day, write them down, otherwise you may forget to do something.

3) Use association with new information, or ask yourself how the information relates to ideas you are already familiar with. Try familiar stimulus such as repeating or grouping similar ideas. Focus on areas of your life that you are passionate about such as family or friends, gardening, working around the house, cooking, etc. Take a selected area such as gardening, for example, and expand on it in your mind. Think about certain flowers or plants you would like to plant and why particular plants or flowers would enhance your landscape. Would these new plants look good with other plants or flowers already planted in a certain area, or will the location be more conducive to their survival. Try to think deeply about your decision and write down your thoughts. Writing these thoughts down will allow you to focus more intently on them and aid in coming up with more ideas about them.

4) Explain your new idea to someone else in your own words. This is a great tool for increasing memory because you are remembering through teaching. Take the gardening idea above. Once you have all your ideas written down and more organized in your mind, explain your ideas to family members. Ask for their input on the subject to help you come up with even more ideas.

5) Don't worry about what others think when you think out loud. Recite what you are reading or review notes out loud. When someone writes you a letter, read it out loud to yourself or to a family member. When you see news flashes scrolling across the bottom of the TV screen read these out loud to yourself. When cooking from a recipe, read the recipe out loud.

6) After learning something new, make time to review the information. Retention is accomplished by review, so remember this phrase and it will help you to remember to review. A good example of this would be preparing a new dish from a recipe. After you prepare it the first time, review the recipe several times in an attempt to commit it to memory and try to prepare it from memory the next time without using the recipe. Keep in mind that this is merely an exercise so if you don't remember all the ingredients, don't hesitate to refer to the recipe. The more you force your mind to remember the better and the more often you use this process the better.

7) Exercise your memory as often as possible. Learn a new subject or re-learn an old subject from your past schooling, such as math, science, history, or something you have forgotten. I remember how much I hated history when I was in school, and as a result did not excel in the subject. Now history it is extremely interesting to me and I enjoy all aspects of the subject. As a result, I exercise my mind with this subject quite often. There are so very many ways to exercise your memory by thinking of the things that interest you personally the most and then channeling your focus in these areas. Another example for me personally is writing. I enjoy very much picking a subject that interests me and writing about it. This is an awesome way to exercise your memory.

8) Keep a journal to exercise the mind. It will also help you to remember through review. With regard to my last example above, whether you write in a journal, work on a book, write poetry, or letters to loved ones and friends, do it on a daily basis. Try to set aside a certain time each day for writing and stick to this schedule.

9) Do crossword puzzles or take advantage of a companion to play board games such as chess, checkers, scrabble, monopoly, etc. since they are excellent exercises for memory. They will help you remember and also sharpen your wit.

10) Practice using visual imagery by going through the steps of actually building something in your mind. If you enjoy working with your hands there are many different things to focus on in this area. I enjoy carpentry work so I am always building something, whether it is a room addition onto our home or a birdhouse. In order to build something, I always first think about what I want it to look like in my mind. If you like to sew, think about what you would like the item to look like and then break down the pattern in your mind. It makes no difference what you enjoy doing as long as you think through the process first and get an image in your mind of what you want the final result to look like. Next, break down the final result into stages in your mind and focus on stage one. This is another great exercise for your memory. For more information from Dr. Blaylock on how to save your brain visit the web site, where you can subscribe to the Blaylock Wellness Report, https://www.newsmaxstore.com/news-letters/blaylock/offer2a.cfm.

You should also do a good thorough Google search for the disease and those who are fighting the battle to find a cure. You, or another member of your family, or friends should assist a loved one or someone you care about, who already has Dementia, by using the ten steps above. Attempt to get them to perform these steps especially in the early stages of the disease to help slow down the degenerative process.

In addition to exercising the brain, there is very strong

evidence that good physical exercise can be very effective in reducing or slowing down the degenerative process in the brain. Researchers have determined that memory, concentration, and abstract reasoning among older adults can be improved by exercising and may even delay the onset of Alzheimer's. Aerobic exercise increases blood flow to the brain, which in turn nourishes brain cells and allows them to function more effectively. A recent study showed that exercise actually promotes the growth of neurons (brain cells) in the hippocampus (the part of the brain that controls memory and learning). According to Waneen Spirduso, Ed.D., a professor at the University of Texas at Austin, and author of "Exercise and Its Mediating Effects on Cognition (Human Kinetics, 2007)," you can get cognitive benefit from as little as walking 20 minutes a day.

Certain nutrients present in some foods are believed to be protective to the brain. Antioxidants in fruits and vegetables have been linked to improved cognitive function. Many types of berries seem especially beneficial in keeping brains spry. James Joseph, director of the neuroscience lab at the USDA Human Nutrition Research Center on Aging at Tufts University says that they have found that the berry fruits improve neuronal communication. The Alzheimer's Association recommends colorful fruits like berries, raisins, prunes, oranges, and red grapes. They also recommend a diet high in dark colored vegetables like kale, spinach, beets, and eggplant. You should be aware of the fact that fish like salmon or trout, are high in heart healthful omega-3 fatty acids. If something is good for the heart, it is naturally good for the brain.

There are some very good games and computer software available to help stimulate and improve brain function. Most of these programs and games do not stipulate that they will help the brain in this way, however one does. BRAIN FITNESS PROGRAM (www.positscience.com) is the only commercial software that is backed up by published research suggesting that it actually enhances brain function. This software involves the user to wear headphones and use a computer to perform audio exercises. This program costs $395.00 for one user and $495.00 for two. MINDFIT (www.mindfit.com) is a PC software that offers exercises to improve short-term memory, reaction time, eye-hand coordination, and more. The cost of this game is $139.00 for the download or $149.00 for the CD for one user. There is an additional cost of $99.00 for each additional user. BRAIN AGE (www.brainage.com) is a game for Nintendo's hand-held DS system that offers 15 different puzzles and exercises plus 100 Sudoku puzzles. The cost for this game is $19.99. BIG BRAIN ACADEMY (www.bigbrainacademy.com) is a game for Nintendo's Wii or DS hand-held systems. In this game, up to eight players can compete in a myriad of activities. These activities include such things as memorization, math problems, and matching shapes to pictures. The cost for this game is $49.99 for Wii, or $19.99 for DS. MY BRAIN TRAINER (www.mybraintrainer.com) is a web site that offers 39 exercises for the brain and charges $29.95 for one year. RADICA BRAIN GAMES and BRAIN GAMES 2 (www.radicagames.com) are hand-held games that offer exercises asking you to complete sequences, find hidden words, solve math problems and more. Dr. Gary Small, renowned neuroscientist and author of *The Memory Bible*, developed a device called The Handheld Brain and Memory Fitness Trainer. It contains five brain exercise games that can improve brain and memory efficiency. This handheld device has an easy-to-read LCD and the included games are Sequence, Mind Game, Flash Card, Word Hunt, and Word Recall. These games simultaneously exercise the left brain (verbal memory and logical skills) and the right brain (visual memory) while automatically tracking your progress. This game also includes a paperback copy of *The Memory Bible* and sells for around $30.00. Lumosity, a brain training program consisting of engaging brain games and exercises developed by some of the leading neuroscientists in the country is also available at this web site, https://www.lumosity.com/sign_up/new. The use of this game can be purchased on a month by month basis for $9.95 per month. If you purchase the use of it for an entire year it is about $6.65 per month. Card games, board games and picture puzzles that aren't too complicated can also improve memory function. All of these games require thought processes to play. Anything you do to keep your brain functioning at as high a degree as possible should have a positive effect.

Also check out all the medications available and quiz their doctor about each of them. Keep the doctor informed of their progress or the lack of it in the interest of whether or not he or she feels the medication prescribed should be changed. You should stay on top of any new medication that comes available for the benefit of your loved one since your doctor may not. If you hear of something new, find out what their doctor and even some other doctors think of the new medicine's potential for your loved ones situation. Since Dementia refers to a group of diseases, there are several different medications that may be prescribed by your doctor. The exact medication they select depends on several factors including the specific type of Dementia your loved one has, as well as their present stage of the disease. Some people, including my mother, have had promising results while taking a combination of these medications simultaneously. We had my mother on a combination of

Aricept and Namenda for about three years, and we firmly believe that she would have been further along in the degenerative process if it were not for the use of these two drugs together. Since everyone's needs are different, you must thoroughly discuss with your doctor what would be the best course of action for your loved one.

Foot note: Be advised that any product prices mentioned may vary depending on when or where you attempt to purchase them.

Foot Note, James Joseph, director of the neuroscience lab at the USDA Human Nutrition Research Center on Aging at Tufts University

Foot Note, Waneen Spirduso, Ed.D., professor at the University of Texas at Austin.

Foot Note, The Blaylock Wellness Report

Chapter 3
BECOMING AWARE OF THE FIRST SIGNS OF DEMENTIA

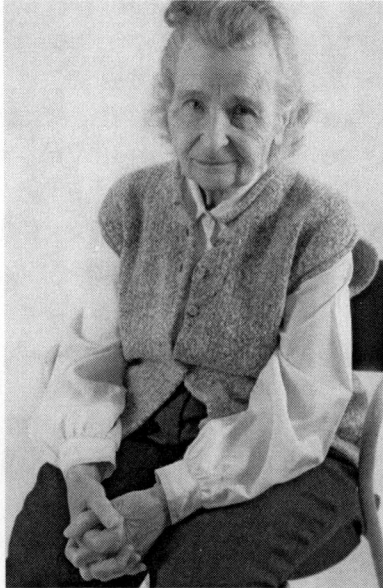

If you suspect that your loved one may have Alzheimer's disease or some form of Dementia, it is extremely important that you act quickly and have them checked out specifically for any form of Dementia. You should contact the Alzheimer's Association (800-272-3900) and ask them for the name of a geriatric dementia specialist. You will also want to find out where the closest dementia diagnostic center is located because they will have the most current information available on Dementia and Alzheimer's. You may wish to go to a specialist that you know can diagnose the early stages of this disease and bypass their personal physician. Early diagnosis is critical because there are a few medications available that will slow the progression of the disease in most people and there by pro-long the need for a full time caregiver. Obviously, if they do have the disease, the sooner they get on medication, the better. You should realize that depression can also display Dementia-like symptoms so this is why taking your loved one to the best possible doctor is so very important. It is critical to get an accurate diagnosis on their first examination.

It would be such a waste to assume that your loved one was merely in a severe state of depression and spend valuable time dealing with this as the issue instead of the real problem. The period of time spent dealing with the depression issue prevented your loved one from getting on desperately needed medication at the earliest possible time.

When a loved one has Alzheimer's disease or other forms of Dementia, there are many things you will begin to notice. Some of these things will be modest things at first, or small changes in their behavior, or attitude, or mental capability. As time goes on, the things you noticed first will worsen and you will begin to notice more changes in other things they do as well. As their condition worsens even further, there comes a time when family and friends have to take it on themselves to intervene and affect the loved one's everyday life for their own safety. One very important thing to learn very early on is that you cannot reason with a person with Dementia. They no longer have the capability of in-depth understanding or the ability to think things through to a resolve or solution. It is for this reason that it will be fruitless to try to explain why something they are doing is wrong. They have lost their ability to rationalize. This was one of the hardest things for us to grasp in the beginning since mother had

LIVING ALONE WITH DEMENTIA—ALZHEIMER'S

always been so easy to talk to and reason with. She always had total confidence in us and interested in our opinion. Another thing that becomes totally necessary as a trade off for their safety is that you have to learn to tell them little white lies and do it often. You can think of these as love lies, health lies, prescription lies or what ever you want to call them but the bottom line is that they are a very necessary part of their care. Regardless of whether this goes against your grain or not, if you want to deal with all the problems that will arise and allow them to maintain their illusion of individuality and self-respect, you have to do it. If you realize the need to take away their car or their cooking ability, for example, for safety reasons you can't just steel it from them or take it away from them for no good reason, or they will rebel and turn against you and then you've lost their trust. One of the most important things to remember is to try to retain their trust through out the entire disease process. You will need to rely on their trust in you for many hurdles that will have to be overcome. If they trust what you tell them, they will tend to do what you tell them and believe that it is in their best interest. They may argue with you a bit from time to time, but in the end they will more than likely see things your way if handled properly. If you lose their trust, they will be argumentative and defiant at every hurdle, and life will be miserable for everyone involved. It is so easy to get off on the wrong foot with them in the early stages of their disease because some of the things they do or say will be aggravating and annoying. They may, at certain times, be just plain nasty or belligerent, or harshly criticize you. In most cases, this is just another hurdle and is totally over a specific issue that can be resolved. Eventually they will forget about it completely. Since everyone is different, there will be certain hurdles with some people that will be more difficult and require more creativity to overcome than others. Getting the car away from some individuals will be more difficult than others, while the checkbook problem could be less challenging for some than others. Try to remember these are just temporary hurdles. I firmly believe that one thing that was helpful in our case was that one of the three of us, (my two sisters and I) needed to be the good guy. My sisters allowed me to play out this role. There were times when it was necessary to be more forceful about a certain issue than others. After several attempts to convince our mother to stop doing certain things failed, one or the other of my two sisters would have to be more forceful. They would have to push her on these issues to get her to come around, sometimes to the point of turning her against them temporarily. My role as the good guy was to re-enforce what they were trying to get her to do by constantly building up their good intentions to my mother, and how much they loved her. By me remaining the good guy, she always felt like she had a confidant and it was through this role that I was able to assist my sisters in accomplishing what we needed to accomplish. I would never push her to the point of getting mad at me because I needed her to believe what ever I told her. I believe you should give in to them in a discrete way regarding minor issues in the early stages of the disease as often as you can so they feel they still have some control in their life. There is a fine line here between letting them do some of the minor things they want to do that are safe for them but without loosing credibility with them. You want them to be able to hold on to their individuality and self-respect so they don't feel like giving up on life, but at the same time you want them to respect what you tell them. You have to maintain their confidence in your opinion and your recommendations so before criticizing something they are doing, think it through and decide if you can leave this issue alone for a while longer. You have to remember that it is not them, but the effect of this terrible disease on them that makes them do or say some of the things they say and do. When you are with them, always treat them as though they are the same loved one they have always been and don't let them know you are aware of their disease. Try to always come across as loving and caring with their best interest at heart.

There are several different symptoms of Dementia and some are quite obvious and some not so obvious. Some of these symptoms apply to specific types of Dementia, and some are only obvious at certain stages of the disease. We will discuss most of these in more detail later.

They develop memory loss that progressively gets worse, a decreased ability to solve problems, inferior judgement skills, and a greater state of confusion. They become hallucinogenic or delusional, and their perception is altered. An inability to recognize familiar people or objects or recognize certain things through their senses becomes a problem.

Their sleep patterns change, motor skills become awkward, and they become disoriented at times and develop a Lessened capability to learn.

They become unable to rationalize and develop Short and long term memory loss with varied language problems as well as becoming unable to read and/or write. A wide variety of personality changes become obvious and they become unable to care for them selves, which leads to a decreased interest in life in general.

Foot Note, Alzheimer's Association web site

Foot Note, Jacqueline Marcell, Eldercare / Alzheimer's Speaker, Author, Radio Host, Caregiver Advocate

Chapter 4
GETTING YOUR LOVED ONE INTO A CLINICAL STUDY

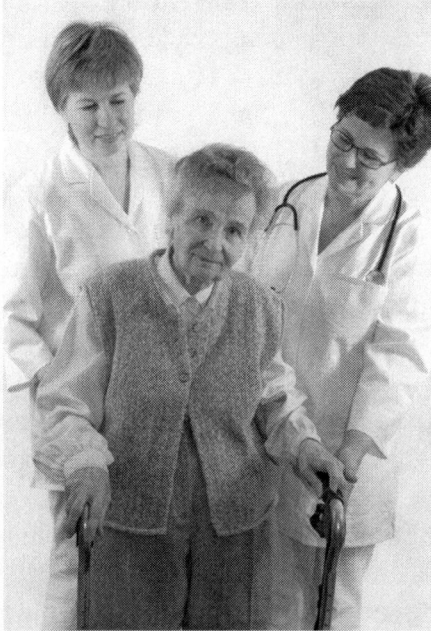

Over the past few years, scientists have made great strides in determining the affects on the brain of various types of Dementia. They have learned much to help with promising new strategies for treating, preventing, and diagnosing the disease. A large number of these studies have been performed on laboratory animals but after many successful studies on animals, it becomes necessary at some point to do clinical studies. These clinical studies are studies on human volunteers. There are over 150 studies going on presently in need of participants who may or may not have memory loss problems or Alzheimer's disease.

There are several reasons why you should consider these clinical studies. Any newly considered treatment has great promise and is considered to be potentially as good or better than the therapies currently available. Since there are no known cures at the present time, any thing new still has the possibility of being something closer to a cure than where we presently are. Most of these studies are at no cost to the patient other than the travel expense of getting back and forth. If your loved one is selected for one of these studies, not only are they closely monitored and supervised, but also they are getting in on the ground floor of the potential benefit of the study. If you think back to the previously mentioned statistics on how many people have the disease and are likely to get it, you must acknowledge the importance of doing anything and everything to assist with developing a cure. Participants involved in these studies receive a very high standard of care. If you choose to participate in one of these studies, assuming you are approved to do so, you are also helping scientist fight the diseases for the benefit of others as well as yourself.

If you are interested in applying for one of the available studies, visit this web site, http://www.alz.org/ alzheimers_disease_clinical_trials_index.asp or contact the Alzheimer's Association at 1-800-272-3900.

Foot Note, Alzheimer's Association web site

Chapter 5
YOU BEGIN TO NOTICE
MEMORY LOSS

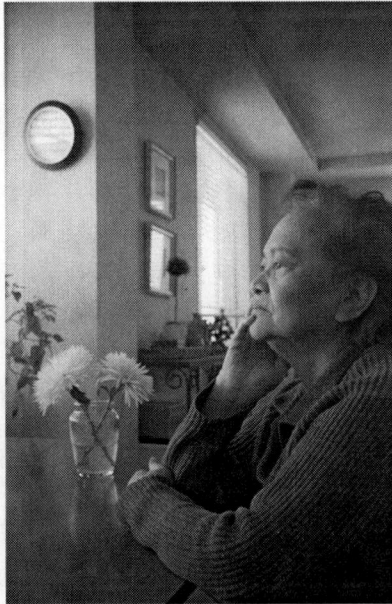

They will begin to develop a degree of memory loss at first that will affect them in many different areas of their life. People they use to know will sometimes seem to be strangers to them. As time goes by, this will become much worse and they will even forget certain family members and close friends at times. Also they will acquaint total strangers with their childhood or other periods in their life, or imagine relationships that did not exist. A good example would be someone on television; to them, they may appear as someone who lived across the street from them when they were growing up. There were two different individuals on TV that my mother would claim lived across the road from her grandma Brown when she was very young. One of these individuals was Tiger Woods. Both of them are actually very young now and my mother was 86 years old. She would comment on what fine young men they had become. Yet Tiger Woods, the famous golfer, did not live across the street from her grandmother nor is he old enough to have lived back when my mother was very young. Your loved one may ask what happened to a relative who has been dead for years. In my mother's case, she would from time to time ask what happened to her mother and daddy, who passed away over 30 years ago. She would ask if her television was her mother and daddy's or would ask when I had seen them. On one occasion, my sister took my mother to the doctor. Later that same afternoon, my mother asked if her mother had gone with her to the doctor. She would constantly ask when we had been over to see her mother and daddy. She would forget such things as her sister having cancer, even though her sister, who has since past away, had cancer for over nine years at that point. She would ask why we failed to tell her that she was sick. When trying to answer your question, or talk to you, words they attempt to use escape them. It's so obvious that they are trying so hard to reach for a particular word but they end up having to settle for one that may or may not be appropriate to the conversation. My two sisters took my mother to visit her sister, who was in an assisted living facility at the time. My mother had not seen her sister in several weeks, yet after saying hello, she had little else to say the rest of their time there. She simply lacked the ability to participate in meaningful conversation any longer. It's really difficult to understand how they could forget to do things such as put their false teeth in to eat, or put their glasses on to see, or put on their hearing aid to hear, but they will do all of these things at times. I would catch my mother trying to eat without her false teeth in, and trying to watch TV without her glasses or her hearing aid. She had to have both in order to comfortably see and hear. My mother was a wonderful cook all her life, but she began to forget to include certain ingredients for items she had cooked from memory thousands of times before. She would forget how long to cook something, or start preparing something and forget that she was even doing it. We began to notice a distinctive difference in the way things tasted compared to how wonderful the same items used to taste. Eventually only the basic functions of a TV remote become possible for them. By this I mean that they merely are able to turn the TV on or off or adjust the volume, and even this becomes a problem at some point. The memory loss is a tough problem for us to accept, especially when we are forced to realize that the day will come when they will forget who we are as well. This is already a problem for us at times. Occasionally my mother will ask me if I am her brother or ask one of my sisters if they are her cousins. Other times she would seem to know exactly who we were and would even refer to our spouse by name and asks how they were doing.

There will be times when they are trying to refer to an item such as a TV screen, the telephone, the mail, newspaper, or it could be anything and they have to refer to these items as something other than what they are. The correct name for these items simply escape their memory. If you ask if they have had dinner, they may say they have even though in actuality they haven't. This could be because the word dinner means something totally different to them at that moment. They may think you mean lunch and they may remember eating lunch so this is why they answered yes. More likely, they can't remember whether they had dinner or not, and just offer an answer to your question. Often, I would call my mother in the morning and ask her if she had a good breakfast. She would giggle and remark "no but I just finished a good dinner" as though I was confused about whether it was morning or evening. She seldom knew what period of the day it was any longer.

Try to ask open-ended questions to get more of a response, as often as possible such as "What did you have for breakfast?" instead of "Did You have breakfast?" which requires only a yes or no answer. You could ask, "How do you feel?" as opposed to "Do you feel alright?" since the latter requires only a yes or no answer. Any question that is considered open ended and requires more than simply a yes or no answer will help to stimulate their brain and keep them sharper. There's a book by Cindy O'Neill and her sister Barbara Iderosa entitled "Mothballs in My Attic". The idea is that one word can spark a lot of memories. Their book offers over 200 opportunities to complete the sentence. This would be a great way to help spark conversations with your loved one.

My mother had to take several pills both in the morning and at night. For someone with a form of Dementia, they will become unable to take pills from a bottle or box after a certain point as my mother did. Initially, we purchased a set of pillboxes that allowed us to place her morning pills in the top compartments for each day of a seven-day period, and her evening pills in the bottom compartments for the same seven days. To simplify things for us, we also purchased a second set of these pillboxes so we could have the next week's pills ready to put out to replace the empty set from the previous week. This technique seemed to simplify taking the pills for her at first and she was able to do it on her own, however, soon she could no longer remember to take them. We first started placing little notes around in strategic locations to help remind her to do certain things, such as taking her pills, which helped for a short while. After a while she stopped paying any attention to the notes. I began to call her every night to remind her to take her pills and my sister would call her every morning. There was a period after we began calling her to remind her to take the pills that we would simply remind her and hang up, and then assume she would take them. We soon discovered that even after we called her to remind her, she would often hang up and still forget to take them. We knew this because we would find pills in the boxes that should have been gone but instead were still there. At that point we began to stay on the line until she would go and take them, and then come back to the phone and tell us she had taken them. We also were able to monitor her on camera and actually watch her take them. I will go into this camera system and other electronic equipment available in more detail later.

As I mentioned above, placing notes around the house seemed to help for a short while, but eventually she stopped noticing them. Placing a list of important telephone numbers by the phone seemed to help for a longer period of time though. She did refer to this list of phone numbers and continued to call us when she felt like it. Unfortunately she got to a point where she no longer thought to place a call to anyone, nor did she answer the phone when she was called. We were able to get her a special phone through a program called the Telecommunications Devices Access Program or T.D.A.P. for short. They can be contacted by email at TDAP.TRA@STATE.TN.US, or their phone number is 1-800-342-8359, ext. 179 or 206. Their street address is Tennessee Regulatory Agency, 460 James Robertson Parkway, Nashville, Tennessee 37243-0505. A qualification application must be filled out and sent in along with a letter from the doctor confirming the need for the phone. The phone was provided at no cost to my mother, but has since been returned because she no longer needed it. There are a couple of distinct advantages to the phone, such as bright lights flash when the phone rings and the ring is very loud. Because my mother was so hard of hearing and even forgot to wear her hearing aid much of the time, we felt this phone would be very helpful to her. The bright flashing lights would call her attention to the phone even if she didn't hear it ring. Unfortunately, after a certain period of time, the flashing light meant nothing to her and she completely forgot that she was receiving a phone call when it flashed. The use of this phone did allow us a few more months of being able to call her on the phone. If you feel the need for a phone such as this, you could contact the agency above or seek out an organization within your own city or state that might provide it.

In the advanced stages of Alzheimer's, the memory loss can get so severe that they can forget critical things such as chewing their food or they may chew continually or for longer than necessary. They can forget to swallow and when this occurs, alternative methods of nourishment become necessary. They mumble words or parts of words with no knowledge of what they are attempting to say. You are unable to understand them because they have forgotten how to converse. They tend to sleep a great deal more often than normal. In the event that they become hospitalized, it is almost impossible to get them to attempt to do for themselves to get better because they have lost the knowledge of why this is so important. Its not that they are being lazy or taking advantage of having someone do things for them but instead they have lost the urge for survival. They no longer realize the importance of doing for themselves in an effort to get stronger.

Chapter 6
THEY BEGIN REPEATING THEMSELVES

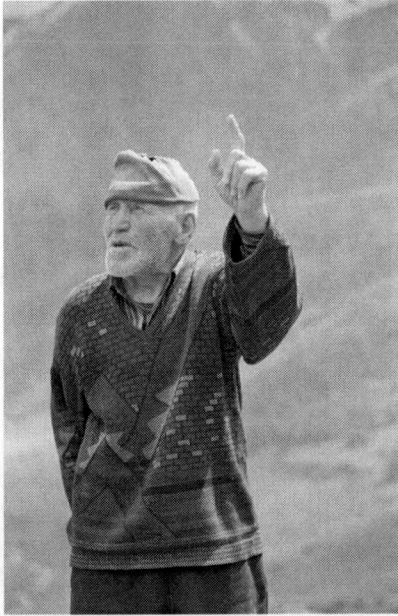

People with Alzheimer's begin repeating the same things over and over, and this only gets worse with time. This situation eventually becomes so extreme that they are no longer able to carry on an intelligent conversation because of it. In time they will begin to talk to themselves a great deal even when others are in the same room with them. I would take my mother a hot lunch and shortly after we finished eating, she would ask if it was time to eat lunch. She would do this several times the remainder of the afternoon. Each time I would simply remind her that we had already had lunch but that I would be glad to fix her something to eat if she was still hungry. In the middle of the afternoon she would ask if I had eaten breakfast. She would do things like this several times through out the same afternoon. One of her grandchildren gave her a small stuffed scarecrow doll and placed it in a hanging plant that hung in the corner of the kitchen. For months whenever any of us were there, she never failed to comment about that doll that someone placed in her plant. Some days she would mention it several times. She did seem to enjoy its presence and it did give her something to talk about. Very often when we would visit her she would mention things that the neighbors had said. On one occasion she was working in her yard and the neighbor's son must have jokingly ask her to marry him and she must have told us this story a hundred times. On another occasion the lady that lived on the other side of my mothers home asked her if the hedge row between their two houses belonged to her or to my mother. My mother was quick to let her know that my dad and her planted that hedge many years ago but here again we heard this story numerous times after that. Her next door neighbor's elderly father died and we must have heard about his passing every time we visited my mother for months afterwards. Constantly bringing up the weather was a subject my mother would use a great deal, or mentioning over and over how bright the sun was. If the sun went behind a cloud, she never failed to mention how gloomy it had become each and every time it occurred. When the situation occurs that they are no longer able to intelligently contribute to a conversation, people who use to call them or visit, might begin to stay away or call less frequently. My mother's cousin would often call to check on her and see how she was doing. My mother would call her back several times later the same day to talk to her without remembering that she had previously called her that day. Naturally this wore on her cousin's patience and so her cousin stopped calling my

LIVING ALONE WITH DEMENTIA—ALZHEIMER'S

mother as often. You can only imagine how annoying this could be unless you were in my mother's cousin's position. This is when people who really care are needed the most. This was a situation where my mother's cousin probably could have avoided all of the return calls by calling to check on her at a time close to her bed time. Mother would not have remembered to call her the next day and her cousin would not have become annoyed. Unfortunately, it's not always that easy to figure these things out in time to implement them. We all have to join together and help to keep their mind as active as possible and constantly consider their degenerative state of mind. The best way to do this is to continue to call them, visit with them, and constantly challenge their memory. Ask them questions about the past, or make comments about the past or family members. Probe their memory to see if you can get them to interject any relative comments or responses. Remember to ask open-ended questions and pass around to other family members the book by Cindy O'Neill and Barbara Iderosa, "Mothballs in My Attic". Choose some open-ended sentences that apply to your loved one, and attempt to get them to complete them.

Go and dig out old family pictures and quiz them on who the subjects are in the photos. My mother still enjoyed looking at photographs until the last weeks of her life but unless they were old photographs, she didn't know who they were. In some of the old photographs, she could still name some of the people in them. Whenever anyone would send my mother a letter, she would read it over and over, not in the same period, but each time with the same degree of interest as the last. She loved to sit and read the news flashes that would scroll across the bottom of the TV screen and she would do it out loud. Reading forces them to recall words and helps to stimulate their mind. Even though we may get nothing from a conversation with them ourselves, we have to realize that we are helping to stir their memory and helping to keep it viable a little longer. This should be the purpose for the call or the visit. Even though they may not even realize whom they are talking to, you must understand that it is the Dementia that has robbed them of their memory and treat them the same way you always have.

Foot Note, Caring Today, November/December 2008, Page 2, *(Things We Like)*

Chapter 7
LOSING THINGS BECOMES A PROBLEM

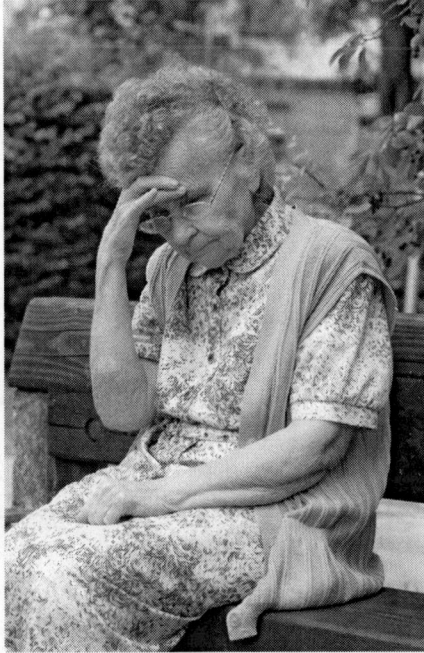

Losing things is another obvious sign you will begin to notice. These may be minor things at first that may or may not get your attention because we all have a tendency to do this from time to time. This will begin to occur more and more frequently however and the items will become more and more major. They will lose important items such as their hearing aid or their glasses or their false teeth. My mother always put her false teeth in a glass on the sink at night, but it got to a point where that glass with her teeth could end up anywhere. Then the teeth would end up in one place and the glass in another. We found her false teeth in a napkin in the dresser drawer on one occasion and in the kitchen cabinet on another. She would sometimes put her hearing aid in different locations and forget where to look for it. Once we found her hearing aid in one of her purses in the dresser drawer. Her situation got to a point where she had to look in several different locations for many things. Very seldom could she get up and go directly to something she wanted. When she would lock her doors from the inside, she would hang a key to a particular door on a nail near the door. She began loosing these keys, because she would forget to hang them back on the nail beside the door, so it became necessary to have several spare keys available just for this reason. There were many items that would end up missing at various times. Articles of clothing would suddenly end up in a different closet from where they should be, or her handbag would get misplaced. Certain kitchen items would suddenly disappear, such as a portable hand mixer, coffeepot, etc. At times she would throw things away for no good reason. Sometimes she would say that something was broken but in actuality it was fine. She had merely forgotten how to use it so she assumed it was broken and threw it away. She would often misplace her TV remote. I remember at our family Christmas get-together last year, we all spent most of that time together looking for mother's TV remote and we never found it. After we went out and purchased another one, the original one turned up a day or two later.

Fortunately, if she does lose the remote, you can purchase a generic remote to replace it in most cases. I might mention that you could also buy an exceptionally large remote so that operating it is easier for them. You can further simplify these remotes by taping over unnecessary buttons that they will not be able to use anyway. They will merely need to be able to turn the TV on and off, and change stations and volume if possible. When their problem of losing things gets so severe that they run the risk of getting lost themselves, you have to take some action regarding their activities. I would suggest that you sign them up with the National Identification Registry, in an area such as the association's Safe Return program. This program can be located on this web site, www.alz.org, and once on their home page, click on the link for MEDICALERT+SAFE RETURN. The importance of this program is that your loved one would have vital emergency information on their person at all times. Should they wonder off and become lost, any responding agency or person who finds them would have the information readily available to them. There would also be a phone number on an ID bracelet they wear that would allow the safe return of your loved one to you.

What you must understand is that when your loved one begins to lose major things on a regular basis, its not going to be long before they will lose themselves unless you, the caregiver take the necessary steps to prevent it. Losing materialistic things is merely a sign of worse things to come. The major losses, besides them getting physically lost themselves are their mental and physical capabilities. These are the losses you must begin to prepare for, because they will surely come. Different people travel down this road at different rates. Some progressively degenerate more slowly than others and merely one of the determining factors are the degree of care the person is able to get. Other factors include the person's age, the type of Dementia they have been diagnosed with, the stage of the disease they happen to be in as well as other health issues the person may have.

Foot Note, www.alz.org, MEDICALERT+SAFE RETURN

Chapter 8
BECOMING DISORIENTED

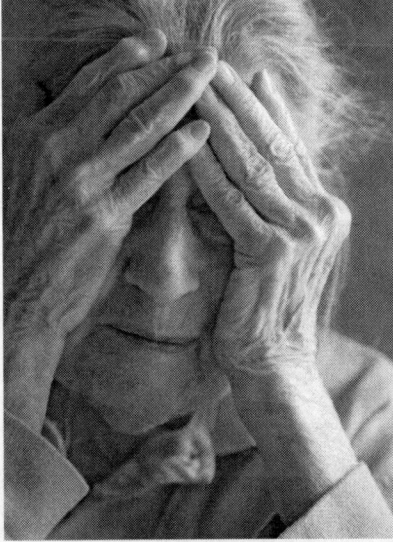

Disorientation becomes a very obvious symptom that gradually worsens. This occurs slightly at first to where they may get up to go to the bathroom and go toward another room instead. Eventually you may return home from having taken your loved one some place and they may ask whose home you are in. When you visit someone else's home and the time comes to leave, they may tell you to come back to see them as though they were in their own home. You have to explain to them that you are taking them with you to their home. One day my mother was sitting on the couch in her living room and about 3:00pm she decided she needed to check and see what she had in the fridge for dinner. She got up and instead of going to the fridge, she went to the bedroom and looked around in a confused manner and stated in a low voice to herself "there's some stuff ". She then opened the bedroom closet door and looked intensely and then remarked again in the same tone, "there's some stuff there". She then opened the guest bedroom door and walked into the guest bedroom and made the same comment, so at this point, I suggested we go to the fridge and check to see what was there and she agreed. Quite often she will get up from her seat and walk into another room with no recollection of why she was doing it. Sometimes she would start to get up and then settle back in her seat, and then start to get up again and then settle back in her seat again all the while with a look of total confusion on her face. When I asked her what she needed, she would in a very confused manner and with that strange look on her face, try to think of what it was that she needed to do. She normally was unable to do so. She gets totally disoriented when she is around several people regardless of whether they are family members or not, or whether the situation was in her own home or not. She finally got to where she only remembered immediate family members and only did that sometimes. She did have several grandchildren, but could no longer remember who they were. At times she would think that other family members who had been deceased for years were still with us. She would often ask when one of them was coming for a visit or wish to know if they were going someplace with her. Although my mother and dad were always very close, she asked on one occasion if my dad left her or in other words walked out on her or divorced her. Of courses he passed away several years ago but we can't imagine where this question came from. Although she could only remember the most immediate of family members at that time, we could get down an old family photo with several family members as children from her childhood and she was still able to name a few of them.

She could name family members from three generation's back occasionally but could not name her own grandchildren. Once when my sister called her, she immediately wanted to know if my sister was going to pick her up and take her to school. The last school she attended was high school many years ago. When this degree of disorientation would occur, we would merely try in a very loving way to explain the actual circumstances or situation that actually existed at the time. We knew that the only way to deal with the underlying cause for this problem was to constantly try to spark her memory in various ways to attempt to keep her memory as sharp as we could for as long as we could. We knew we could not bring back the loss of memory but simply try to slow down the degenerative process. I mention several ways to do this through out these chapters that definitely seemed to help with our case. In spite of all you do, the day will surely come when they no longer realize where they are nor even what time of day or night it is. Their mind will simply no longer seem to wonder about such things. They will no longer care about watching TV or listening to it or the radio. Reading or writing will no longer interest them at all nor even having someone read to them. They will merely seem to enjoy, if enjoy is the proper word, someone's presence in the room. They may make little mumbled comments that are in most cases impossible to understand and occasionally give you a little smile. It is probable that they will constantly talk to themselves in their sleep and sometimes may even laugh out loud in their sleep. We can only wonder and wish we knew what they were thinking at the time.

Chapter 9
FORCING CHANGES ON THEM, BUT DOING IT DISCRETELY

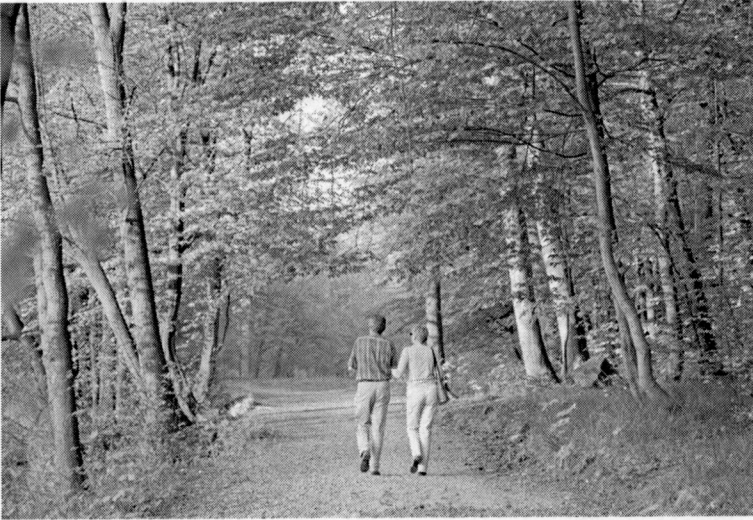

Exercising tough love decisions becomes necessary at many points through out the progression of Dementia and each situation is different and requires serious consideration as to when to implement a change and to what degree. It is so very important to keep everything as simple as possible for them. Any change to their everyday lifestyle should be made with simplicity in mind because everything will only become more and more difficult for them in time. Any situation that presents itself as any type of threat to your loved one must be dealt with as quickly as possible, but if time permits, should be done in such a manner that they are included in the decision process or at least are made to think they are. They may or may not be capable of this degree of input, but at least if discretely handled, you can make them feel like the change was partially their decision. When you begin to determine that a mental disorder such as Alzheimer's exists, immediately consider all the ways that they could accidentally harm themselves and take action, especially regarding certain critical areas. All of the things that should be dealt with as soon as they become necessary are at the discretion of the individual caregiver, while at the same time trying not to create a home that feels too restrictive. The home should encourage independence, meaningful activities, and social interaction. A book worth checking out is entitled "Making Your Home Senior-Friendly" by Chuck Oaks. Chuck is a Certified Aging in Place Specialist, who gives innovative tips on making every room of the house safe and convenient. Many of his tips would be great for your loved one especially if they have Dementia. You may choose to use a variation of his ideas in some cases because of the disease, but at least he makes you aware of the many areas to focus on.

There are always various items about the home that a loved one with Dementia could accidentally trip and fall over. These items include such things as coffee tables, floor lamps, magazine racks, foot stools, flower pots, etc. and should be removed from their normal area of activity. Many of these items also have sharp pointed edges or corners that could also impale them when they fall. Remove any throw rugs that could slip when they put their weight on them or that they could possibly trip over. If small children are in the house from time to time, be especially cautious of toys lying around that could pose a problem. Be sure to remove all of these types of items and make the areas your loved one moves around in as clear and easy to traverse as possible. My mother use to love to watch small children and I think for some individuals, including her, this is really quite therapeutic.

One of the very first problems that arose with my mother that had to be dealt with quickly was her finances. Mother had always contributed to certain charitable organizations. This was fine to a reasonable degree based on her financial capability. She began, however, to write checks to every single political and charitable organization that sent her a request or called her on the phone, many of which were scams. She would write checks totaling seven or eight hundred dollars per month in donations, which was an amount she could not afford to spend. Not realizing at this point that she had Dementia, we tried desperately to make her understand the error in what she was doing, but she continued to do it. My sisters and I began to contact all of the people corresponding with her, as well as those who called her, pleading with them to take her off their mailing lists. Some of these organizations agreed to take her off their list, but explained about the lag time involved with her actually falling off the list even after they process our request. Others would agree to do so but she still received their mailers requesting money. Some of the most difficult requests to stop were the political party donation requests. We tried going through the post office to stop the problem but the postal service explained that there was nothing they could do to prevent them from sending the mailers. We did place her on a do not call list which helped somewhat. The only way we were able to completely solve the problem, however, was to take her checkbook away from her and change her mailing address to a post office box number. To emphasize this, remember there will come a time when you will have to remove their check writing privileges and have their mail go to a post office box so you can monitor what mail they receive. Out of love and respect for your loved one, if possible, you must do this in such a way that they don't feel that you are forcing them to do anything. Here again, you have to incorporate lies in your strategy for overcoming these problems. I can't emphasize this enough. This is an important statement that will apply to almost every change you make to their lifestyle. Naturally when you remove their check writing privileges, someone else will have to take on this responsibility. This is one reason why someone must be designated to acquire a durable power of attorney and a healthcare proxy to be able to handle all of their legal and medical affairs. This person will have to be added to your loved one's checking account and have the ability to write checks for them. This is much more easily accomplished if you can do it while they are still coherent enough to go with you to the bank and sign the necessary documents to add you to the account for check writing privileges. We were able to convince my mother that it would be best to add my sister to the account in the event that she got sick and couldn't write checks. There are several ways to approach getting their checkbook away from them discretely when the time comes, and you may have to try different approaches. We first stopped her mail from being delivered to the house so she no longer received the bills or donation requests. We had all of her mail forwarded to a post office box. The post office initially would forward all of her mail to this box temporarily, giving us an opportunity to contact all of her creditors and utilities informing them of her new post office box address. After this period, the post office would only deliver mail to the post office box that was actually addressed to this box number. From this point on, the only mail that was delivered to her was from people who had been given her new post office box number by us. My sisters and I would take turns checking her post office box and the only mail we would give her would be the occasional magazine or something we thought she might enjoy reading. Once we did this and she stopped seeing the reasons coming in every day to write a check, she began to slowly get used to not writing checks. When she would ask where her checkbook was, we would say she was out of checks and we were waiting for the bank to send new ones. My mother was not accustomed to using a credit card even though she had a couple, so these and all of her other financial information was easy to collect and keep safe. This method worked for us to solve this problem, but she did occasionally become confrontational about the check book issue. In each case we were able to quickly get her mind on something else and eventually got passed it.

If your loved one is use to using a credit card, explain that the bank notified you that someone had attempted to steel their identity and they recommended the cards be temporarily cancelled. You should then collect the cards and proceed to cancel them. Explain what a growing problem this is now a day for everyone. Also re-assure them that you are going to take good care of their finances for them from now on. You may or may not be able to easily slide into this role at this point but you are surely laying the groundwork. It shouldn't take long for them to forget about this issue. Once they stop writing checks or using their credit cards, it should be merely a matter of time before they forget that they ever did it in the first place. As bad as it may sound, the memory loss aspect of Dementia does work to your advantage in solving many of the other problems that arise with the disease. The draw back to this is the fact that you will ultimately come face to face with this very major characteristic of the disease and be forced to deal with all the other problems associated with it.

It is extremely important that you or another family member be designated to acquire a durable power of attorney for the benefit of making any and all legal decisions on your loved ones behalf, and a healthcare proxy for medical problems that might arise. There will most certainly come a time when they will be unable to make these decisions on their own. Be sure to get the proper power of attorney to cover all your needs. You should be aware that a general power of attorney would not suffice for both legal and medical needs. Refer to chapter 13 and check out the available helpful resources listed there. Keep in mind that with regard to any legal or medical problems, always research what applies in your own state by seeking legal guidance.

You should keep a unique list of all pertinent emergency telephone numbers handy on your person but at the home as well. These should include everyone you can think of that might be needed to respond in any type of emergency related to your loved one. It is also helpful to have any phone numbers that your loved one calls regularly and any others you feel they may need on a large list by the phone. This list should be readily assessable to them. At some point the list will no longer be necessary, but you want it available just in case they have a temporary memory surge and need one of the numbers.

If they still drive a vehicle, you must start thinking of a way to stop this activity. It will merely be a matter of time before they will forget where they are going or how they got there or how to get home. They may even forget how to negotiate traffic and subject themselves to a terrible accident. The car is one of the first considerations because you want to use discretion to get them out of the vehicle. This is a major life change for most people and not an easy hurdle to overcome. The best way to approach it is while you still have time on your side and can take gradual steps to get them out of the vehicle. There are several things to try and you, as the caregiver must make the final call as to what most likely would work for your particular situation. You may wish to take them to their doctor for an examination and ask that their eye sight, hearing and reflexes be checked. Discretely talk to the doctor without the patient present and explain the situation. If the doctor feels that they should no longer be driving, ask him or her for a letter to that effect. You will want to mail this letter to the Department of Motor Vehicles in an attempt to have their license revoked. The letter from the doctor would also be your excuse for why they have to relinquish their license. This method may require a little time to accomplish, but it might work for you if time is on your side, or if you trust them to drive a few days longer. Someone could possibly transport them during this waiting period without them suspecting anything. If time is not on your side and you need to get them out of their vehicle quickly, you could call the Department of Motor Vehicles and speak with a supervisor explaining the situation. Set up an appointment to take your loved one in for an exam. You should explain to your loved one that apparently someone reported them driving recklessly or possibly speeding but that the DMV is requiring you to bring them in for a routine exam. You are primarily doing this in order to get the DMV to retain their license. If the DMV does suspend their driving privileges, be as supportive as possible and assure them that you will make sure that they will always be able to go where ever they need to go. Continue to reassure them whenever the subject comes up that they will not be homebound, and will have transportation whenever they need it. Naturally you will have to discretely manipulate when these needs actually exist, keeping in mind that the more you can allow them to get out of the house the better. These first couple of ideas, I learned from a very good book entitled *Elder Rage* by Jacqueline Marcell, Eldercare / Alzheimer's Speaker, Author, Radio Host, and Caregiver Advocate.

Try to figure a way to let it be their idea. In my mother's case, we first disabled the vehicle so it would not start. If your loved one is mechanically inclined, this method may not work for you, but in my mother's situation, this was not the case. When she persisted about why we couldn't get it fixed, we explained that there was a very difficult part to acquire on order for it. Another method is to replace their car key with one that looks similar but won't start the car. Try what ever works best to buy you some time for them to forget. Our tactic bought us enough time for her to get use to not driving it, yet she still knew she had a car and that was important to her. During this time, my two sisters and I filled in and did everything for her that she normally used her car for. Eventually she disassociated the need to drive the car for the things she had used it for in the past. At this point it was time to try to get the car completely away from her. Out of sight, out of mind seamed to be the order of the day. Her granddaughter had been driving an old car back and forth to work that was really unreliable and unsafe, so we explained this situation to mother and coaxed her into coming up with the idea of giving her car to her granddaughter. The way we handled it, it was actually my mother's decision, which was very important to her, and she felt good about helping out her granddaughter. So get the car away from them but try to let it be their choice, bearing in mind that the car has to go regardless of how it has to unfold.

A large number of the elderly have full time or part time jobs or hobbies involving the operation of certain types of machinery. Operating machinery will soon become something that will be more and more hazardous for them depending on the type of machinery of course. Steps should be taken to remove this type of activity from their capabilities before it becomes dangerous for them. I'm afraid, at this point they will no longer be able to perform a job. If they are still employed, you will have to explain the circumstances to their employer if they haven't already become aware of the situation. Once you realize they have Dementia, it is advisable to start working to wean them off of any machinery or other equipment that is unsafe for a child. Unfortunately, before very long, they will become childlike in many ways. Sometimes getting them to stop using a piece of machinery may be a difficult hurdle to overcome, but be discrete and subtle when possible and try to convert their interest to something safer. Often, one of the best ways to deal with this problem is to simply disable the machine, if you have this control, and stall them as to why it has not been repaired, until they forget about it. You can say a part for the machine has been ordered but is on back order and will take a while to arrive. This should give you enough time for them to forget about it. Keep in mind that someone with Alzheimer's forgets things much faster than someone without a degenerative brain disorder.

Many elderly people are very athletic and this lifestyle is very important to them. Some things are much more dangerous than others naturally so based on their activities, you should either monitor or cause some degree of change as necessary. If their dementia has affected their motor skills, and eventually it will, they should not be hunting, fishing, camping, horseback riding, snow skiing, water skiing, or anything comparable without close supervision. They should definitely not be allowed to do any of these things alone. The use or handling of firearms should strictly be prohibited, nor should a firearm even be in the home if they live alone. Any sport or other activity that involves any degree of danger should be stopped as soon as possible. Try to get them interested in doing something else athletic, but something they could do with someone. Have some options to offer them before you confront them about ceasing their present activity. Provide them with something else they might like to do before forcing them to give up something they are passionate about.

In all homes there are many dangerous items that have to be removed or at least placed out of reach for safety reasons. Some items are much more dangerous than others especially items such as knives or any sharp pointed objects, small portable appliances such as hand held mixers, blenders, electric skillets, etc. A good rule of thumb might be to ask yourself if you would trust your two year old child with the object and if the answer is no, remove it.

To prevent your loved one from being accidentally burned from over heated water, adjust the hotwater thermostat to 120 degrees or less. They may accidentally burn themselves without realizing it. Safety eventually becomes a non-issue for them so this totally becomes the care givers responsibility.

You will certainly at some point restrict the use of electrical appliances, but until you do, be particularly cautious of any appliance located near a water source. If this situation does exist anywhere, immediately remove it. Do not allow the use of any electrical appliance near water for their sake as well as yours. Water is a great conductor of electricity and you could easily get shocked or even electrocuted.

If they still cook, you will eventually have to wean them off of using the range or eventually they may catch the house on fire. There are many dangers associated with using the range and other kitchen appliances. If they were use to doing a great deal of cooking, this will be another difficult problem to solve but it has to be done. My mother would accidentally leave a towel or potholder too close to an electric eye or leave an eye turned on or leave the oven turned on. She would put food in the oven or on the eye and forget she was cooking. We handled this in much the same way as we handled the car situation. I disconnected the range so she would be unable to use it at all. We explained to her that the range was so old that it wasn't worth repairing even though it wasn't that old. We kept telling her that we were trying to find a new range that had a number of new safety features on it but they were hard to find. This seemed to pacify her and in the mean time we were getting her use to using the microwave for the cooking that she really needed to do. We did go out and get her the simplest microwave we could find for her to operate. Because of her declining memory problem, during this period she forgot all about cooking things from scratch that she used to cook. My sisters and I began taking her hot meals or pre-cooked food whenever we visited her so she always had plenty of freshly cooked food available. This was another large hurdle that we had overcome, so remember to wean them off of using the electric range as soon as possible. Then begin to wean them off of all the other appliances, or install safety features on them such as automatic shut-off switches. I'm afraid at this point it becomes necessary to consider an in-home sitter or at least someone to come in to provide their meals. Mother got to a point where she would simply eat a cold sandwich or bowl of cereal for every meal, unless we were there with a hot meal. This is also when we began to look for a part-time in-home sitter.

Since someone with a mind disorder will at some point

be unable to distinguish between good food and spoiled food, you must regularly keep the refrigerator cleaned out. Be sure that only fresh food is available in the refrigerator at all times. Attempt to keep the items they use more often up front, making these more readily available.

All artificial fruit and any toxic plants should be removed because they may appear to be edible and your loved one could accidentally poison themselves. A large number of the artificial items available today look so much like the real thing, it's quite difficult to distinguish the difference. Someone with Dementia will eventually be unable to distinguish between what should be consumed and what should not.

Naturally in all homes there are many cleaners, paints, and other toxic chemicals that should no longer be available to your loved one. They may easily confuse these items with something to drink and consume something they shouldn't. All of these type items should be locked away, completely out of view.

The use of alcohol is a topic that is strictly an individual caregiver's option to control based on their knowledge of the individual. Just remember that the bottom line is that you must control their alcohol use. Alcohol should not be taken at all with medication or in a close proximity to taking any medication. The patient should be weaned off of alcohol completely as time goes by because they will begin to lose both mental and motor skills on their own and the use of alcohol will only make a bad situation worse.

To prevent your loved one from being able to accidentally lock themselves in a room, such as the bathroom, remove these inside locks. Make sure that no inside doors that are used can be locked on either side unless they lead to an off-limits area, which should stay locked at all times anyway.

My mother had a tile bathroom floor and throw rugs. Unfortunately we failed to catch this problem before she slipped and fell due to this situation. Fortunately we were monitoring her on an electronic camera system when we saw the results of her falling. Luckily for her, we noticed her hand extended out through the bathroom door at floor level. We realized she had fallen and immediately got someone there. We should have carpeted the bathroom floor and any other slippery floor that she could possibly slip and fall on such as a tile or linoleum kitchen floor. You could also paint certain concrete floors with a type of grip guard covering or use certain types of grip guard tape to prevent falling in bathtubs, and showers.

Medications have to be carefully monitored because they will become unable to remember to take their medication, but on an occasion when they do remember, they may take the wrong thing or too many of the correct pills. Due to other health issues, they may be taking certain medications that are critical to their well being and cannot afford to miss taking them without severe consequences. Always be aware that this is one of the most important controls for you to strictly enforce.

You should carefully monitor the use of heating pads and electric blankets to make sure they don't use them in close proximity to any water and also to be sure they don't burn themselves by having too much heat on them for too long a period of time. They will be unable to regulate this process at some point.

As time goes by they will become more prone to get up and wander about the house at night or during the day for no reason. By using illuminated light switches, they will be a little more likely to turn on a light and less likely to fall in the dark when they do wander about.

Because of the tendency to get up and wander or go from the bedroom to the bathroom more often, it would be helpful to install night-lights. Place these wherever you feel necessary but especially between the bedroom and bathroom. By doing this, even if they should fail to turn on a light, they still should be able to see their way.

Under normal circumstances with age comes a greater need for orthopedic assistance devices such as grab bars, support rails, wheel chairs, walkers, walking canes, etc. When they are elderly and have Dementia, their needs become much greater because of the loss of motor-skills. They will begin to fall more and more often. Naturally the more often this happens, the greater their chances of doing themselves some serious harm. At this point the need for a grab bar for them to pull themselves up from a sitting position or to stabilize themselves while standing becomes necessary. Encourage them to begin using a walker, preferably one with wheels, since these are much easier for them to use. There are some walkers with small wheels, but they are not as easily used as those with larger rubber wheels. You can also find a walker that has a seat that would allow them to stop walking and sit to rest if they become exhausted. These are a little more costly but may be quite helpful depending on how much they walk.

All activities eventually become difficult, but standing for a period of time necessary to take a shower can be impossible and a shower seat might be required, or an orthopedic commode seat may be necessary to make going to the restroom easier. Orthopedic commodes sit higher off the floor than regular commodes and make getting up from a sitting position much easier. Making a shower available to them as opposed to a bathtub would be advisable when possible. It's much easier on them to stand or sit on a shower seat than to have to sit down in a bathtub and then get up from this sitting position. Keep in mind, it's all about making their life easier and as simple as possible.

In time there will be parts of the home that will become more dangerous for your loved one than others. Some of these areas will have to be closed off to them. Areas such as attics, garages, basements, lofts, balconies or any place where they could fall or get their hands on something dangerous should be closed off in some way. You can lock and camouflage doorways with decorative rugs or curtains. Access to other areas could be screwed or nailed shut. Remember, out of sight out of mind. Eventually they will forget these areas are there if they are not using them.

Every home should keep a fire extinguisher handy but it is much more crucial for there to be at least one or more in the home of someone with a mind disorder. No matter how safe you may think the home is for them, they might always do the unthinkable to accidentally start a fire. Naturally the extinguisher is primarily for the caregiver's benefit to use, because the loved one would probably never think to use it in the event of an emergency.

We are all aware of the fact that this day in time, it is unsafe to leave your doors unlocked even when you are home especially for the elderly living alone. Several years ago I installed ornamental steel security doors on my mother's home and handrails on all the steps for safety reasons. After she developed Alzheimer's, the steel security doors were even more important than ever as well as the security system we had installed. She did use both most of the time as long as we reminded her to do so. On a normal day in the wintertime, the only time my mother would venture outside was to go out to get the newspaper in the morning. This was a major part of her normal routine that we eventually had to change since she was getting to where she would forget to lock the door behind her when she re-entered her home, and soon got to where she only occasionally read the newspaper anymore. One thing she would always do was to place a chair under the doorknob of each of the exterior doors at night. Even after she occasionally forgot to lock the doors, she always remembered to place the chair under the doorknob. The bad thing about this was that if an emergency ever occurred and we had to get in, we would have had some degree of difficulty doing so and may have been forced to break out a window or break the door down to get in. As I mentioned previously, she reached the point of losing her keys along with many other things more often. It is important to have extra keys available to everything your loved one has access to such as exterior doors, lock boxes, etc.

It is extremely important, where possible, to have someone living near by your loved one keep a set of keys to their home in case of an emergency. You can always call 911 for assistance, but you have no guarantee of how long it may take for them to arrive. If a nearby family member, friend or neighbor has a key to the house, they can probably get there sooner and without doing damage to the home. Fortunately in my mother's case, she was very close to the neighbors across the street and they were always readily accessible in the event of an emergency.

If your loved one has central heat and air in the home, great! If they have wall or space heaters, or wood stoves, or any type of unsafe gas heat, focus your attention on changing this situation so that it is safe for them. Consider their habits and lifestyle and check out optional heat sources. In my mother's situation, she had wall heaters and some of these were no longer safe for her to use in her state of Dementia. There was too great a chance that she would turn one of them on high and forget about it, or place something in front of one and catch the house on fire. She actually did this in a couple of instances and almost did catch the house on fire. There was one room in a part of the house that she didn't even use in the winter time and kept closed off yet she was still turning that heater on high and leaving it on. On one occasion my sister was there for a visit and walked into this room and there was a chair pulled over in front of the heater with a towel across the back of it. Luckily she arrived when she did or there would have been a fire. This was a room with no water pipes to worry about freezing up or anything that would be affected by simply leaving the heat off all winter long. To solve this problem, we simply disconnected this heater. She never asked about why it didn't work. If she had asked why it didn't work, we would have approached this problem much the same way we did with the range. We would have explained that it was defective and that we were looking for a newer more up-to-date heater for that room that was safer to use. We would have continued to use this same excuse as long as it took for her to forget about it. There was another heater in the guest bedroom that we simply turned that particular breaker off to. This heater had curtains hanging on each side and we were concerned that she might turn it on for no good reason and possibly catch the curtains on fire if she forgot about it. The door always stayed shut to this room as well, so it was unnecessary to heat it. Luckily for us she was not in the habit of turning this heater on, so this presented no problem when we disabled it. Any other heaters in my mother's house were in safe locations, out of the way of her normal routine activities. My sisters and I routinely monitored these heaters to be sure she kept them in a safe position. They were UL approved and had all the updated safety features as well. We monitored these when we were there but also from an electronic camera monitoring system we had installed.

If they are used to taking long walks for exercise, you need to take steps to prevent them from doing this by themselves. There will come a day when they will suddenly be walking and all of a sudden they will be lost.

They will have forgotten how to get home and they will be at the mercy of someone accidentally finding them. This could even be a more severe situation where a search party has to end up looking for them with only hope of finding them before they perish due to bad weather, lack of food or water, or worse. It is important that they continue to get their exercise, so the best way to handle this would be for someone to begin to walk with them if this is possible. If family or friends are unable to do this when the loved one is used to doing it because of work schedules or other commitments, try coaxing him or her into walking at a time when someone can walk with them. If this is still not possible, consider hiring someone to provide this service for the loved one. Remember if they are used to walking and still wish to do so, try to make it happen but with a walking partner only. I will always remember a walk that my great aunt and uncle took several years ago. They both had Dementia and both were walking down the road holding hands with no idea where they were going, how they got there, or how to get home. Luckily someone driving down the road had the good sense to stop and question them since they were a long way from any house. This person picked them up and took them to a local store where they were recognized and the family was contacted. My great aunt and uncle were very fortunate to have been found before it was too late.

Foot Note, Caring Today, November/December 2007, *Things We Like*, Page 2

Foot Note, Jacqueline Marcell, Eldercare / Alzheimer's Speaker, Author, Radio Host, and Caregiver Advocate

Chapter 10
EFFECTS ON THE FAMILY OF SOMEONE WITH DEMENTIA

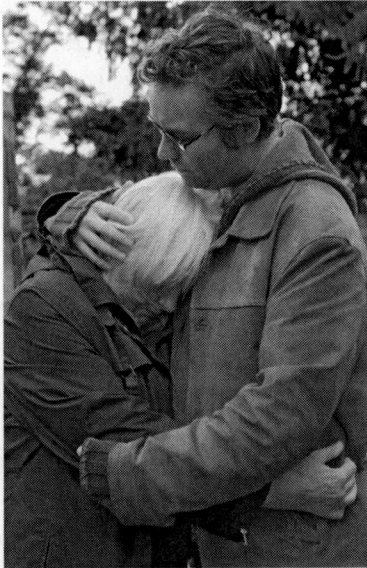

Naturally, going through this period of trying to care for and make life as easy as possible for someone you love who has Dementia, is putting your life on an emotional roller coaster. We are all affected in different ways and to different degrees. One determining factor is how close we are to the individual with the disease. How involved we get with the entire process and how much of our own personal lives we devote to their care plays another big role. Whether or not you have a good strong support system behind you and family who believes in what you are trying to do and how much help you have is very important. You must realize that you can only pour out so much of your heart to someone before you create a void that has to be refilled. Because the person with Dementia will be unable to give this love back to you at some point, you must draw it from the memories of their love and your support system. Remember that your family and friends who are helping share the responsibility through out this process also share a common bond with you. You are all going through the same thing and need to help support each other. If you are unfortunate enough to be going through this period of caring for someone you love with Dementia all alone, seek out a support system. There are several options available to you. First of all contact all of your family members, friends, members of the church, and neighbors, because there may be some help and support there you failed to realize. If for no other reason than your own support system, try to stay as close as possible to family and friends, and lean on them for your own well being. You will need to feel connected during this stressful and trying period. Seek out a support group where you meet others who are caring for a loved one with Dementia. Organizations like the Alzheimer's Association who has a 24-hour help line, 1-800-272-3900, and offices in every state. Their web site is http://www.alz.org/index.asp or contact a local hospital in your area to see if they offer support groups. Find an Alzheimer's Association Memory Walk by visiting http://www.alz.org/memorywalk/overview.asp. These memory walks are for people who have an interest in the fight against this terrible disease.

It is the largest event to help raise awareness and funds for Alzheimer care, support and research. These memory walks are held annually in hundreds of communities across the country, and you can even start your own. You can meet many individuals going through or who have gone through what you are going through. You may even meet someone you know who would be willing to help you in your situation or even someone you don't know who would be willing to help. If it is difficult for you to leave home to attend a support group, go on line and seek out these groups. When you ask for help from anyone, try to ask for specific help, such as someone to sit with your loved one at specific times, or someone to provide them with a hot meal a certain number of times a week or month. Maybe ask for someone to just go by on certain days to check on him or her. Almost anything will help and take a small amount of the pressure off of you. As you acquire people to help and they give you some type of commitment, write these commitments down so you can concentrate on other aspects of their needs as well as your own. Always confirm in some way that these commitments are being fulfilled.

At certain times there may be even greater responsibility on you as a caregiver due to the nature of the disease on your loved one. They tend not to take as good a care of themselves any longer and as a result may develop various infections or other illnesses requiring even more of your time or focus. You may have to spend even more time with them periodically or get others to help you monitor them more closely until this new medical problem is resolved. If they get to a point of no longer being able to maintain balance and begin falling down or falling out of bed at night, you may have to get help. The time has come for someone to be with them 24 hours a day until arrangements can be made for some form of assisted living or a nursing home. This can be an extremely demanding period even with adequate help.

When you are taking care of your loved one you are probably not taking as good a care of yourself as you otherwise would, so your doctor needs to be a part of your support group. You should see your doctor periodically for check ups. Your doctor may see signs of depression or illness in you that you are unaware of. You must remember that you have to remain healthy in order to care for your loved one, not to mention for your own sake.

Foot Note, Alzheimer's Association web site, Memory Walk

Chapter 11

ELECTRONIC DEVICES CAN BE VERY HELPFUL

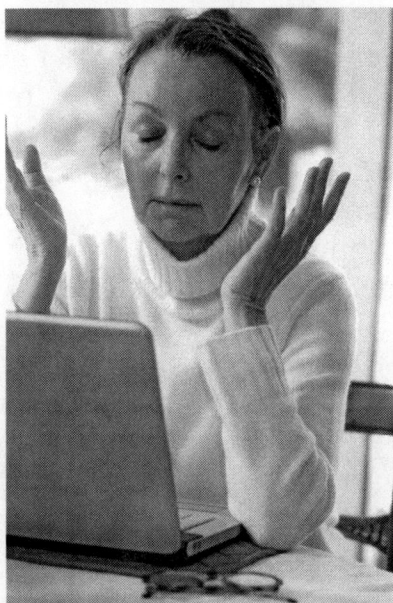

It is most important to have monitored burglar and fire protection for your loved one, especially if they live alone. A reputable company that will immediately notify the local police department should monitor the burglar alarm system. They would also notify you or someone you designate in the event of an emergency. The same system can also be equipped with smoke and heat detectors that would be monitored 24 hours a day, and in the event of a fire alarm, the local fire department would be notified and dispatched as well as yourself or someone you designate. Due to the increased danger of a fire brought on by the degenerative process of the mind of someone with Dementia, this is extremely important. You could check out these systems by contacting ADT Companion Service 1-800-209-7599 or go online to www.adt.com or www.aarp.org/adtcompanion.

Because they will also become more susceptible to falling or hurting themselves, it would also be helpful if they wore an SOS button or a medic alert bracelet or necklace. Either of these devices would allow your loved one to push a button on the device and activate an emergency signal through the existing alarm system. Once the monitoring facility receives the alarm notice, they will notify an emergency service and whom ever else you specify. You should be sure to specify your needs up front when having the system installed. There are many reliable companies, but be sure to check the company out thoroughly that will handle your area to learn about their track record. You can begin your search for this device by contacting ADT at the phone number and/or web site shown above.

There are also pillboxes, pagers, vibrating watches, and dispensers that talk to your loved one or alert you, the caregiver, in the event they forget to take their medication. You can find dozens of options for these devices at E-Pill Medication Reminders (1-800-549-0095) or www.epill.com. They are also available from www.forgettingthepill.com or call them at (1-877-367-4382). These electronic pill boxes, in some cases, will accommodate up to a 30 day supply of pills and alert your loved one up to four times a day to take their pills. The most costly type of electronic pillbox not only reminds the patient when to take the pills but also alerts the caregiver when they fail to take them. If you don't like the idea of loading all the pillboxes, there are other options available. You can set up a service through which your loved one would receive a reminder through a pager, email, phone, or cell phone call, and you as the caregiver could be reminded of certain things as well. These services can also remind them of monthly refill dates, scheduled doctor or dentist appointments, etc.

With my mother's state of mind being what it was and her loss of memory having declined to the state that it had, we began thinking about an in home sitter. This is not an inexpensive undertaking. After doing a bit of research in this area and checking out some other options, we decided the next step should be some electronic monitoring. We figured that some electronic cameras strategically placed in her home that we could monitor from our home computers, in conjunction with our personal visits should suffice for a while longer. My sisters and I stayed in constant touch with each other regarding our mother and we all monitored her several times on any given day. This electronic camera system that we had installed by ADT allowed us to monitor most of her movements with the exception of the bathroom, naturally. It would also allow us to monitor a sitter and know whether we made the correct choice of someone to sit with mother. When my sister or I called her up to remind her to take her pills, we could also observe her taking them. If we saw that she had something too close to a heater, we could call her and discretely get her to move it with out letting her know we were watching her. When we had the cameras installed we decided to tell her that they were motion detectors that we had added to her alarm system. She would never have agreed to being monitored on camera. This was just another little white lie that we had to tell her for her own well being. As I mentioned previously, there were many of these lies that allowed us to deal with so many situations for her best interest. Fortunately my mother had good neighbors who had a key to her house. If we saw that she had fallen or was having some other serious difficulty, we could call them and they could walk right across the street to help her. This is an ideal situation if your loved one falls into this same category with good neighbors. Luckily, mother would still respond positively to suggestions and she would do most anything we suggested. If in the interest of getting her to get a little exercise, we suggested that she get up off the couch and go check to see if the heat was on or check to see if a door was locked, we could watch her do it. This camera system was the greatest thing since sliced bread for someone living alone with Dementia who also has loved ones who care enough to monitor them as we did. I'm sure you can contact most any reputable security company and have one installed. Our system would accommodate four cameras placed where ever we desired with the exception of the bathroom, and we had to be approved to have one installed in the bedroom. Our situation with mother and our reason for wanting to have it installed in her bedroom was acceptable for approval. With the camera strategically placed in her bedroom, we could see her sleeping to be sure she didn't fall out of bed. This camera also was focused straight across her bed down the hall and across her kitchen so we could see a great deal of her activity. We could monitor her getting up to go into the bathroom and even observe the status of two different heaters. The system does require an Internet connection, but if you already have this connection in the home, the camera system itself involves no monthly charge and you purchase the camera system outright. My mothers system, which was a basic system with two cameras but would accommodate four, was approximately $700.00 installed and fully functional. Additional cameras were an additional 235.00 each installed. My sisters and I would merely log on to a web site provided by

ADT, insert our username and password, and monitor her at will. The value of this system to us was that it allowed us to keep mother in her home a little longer without the higher cost of a full time in-home sitter or an assisted living facility which were the next considerations.

Foot Note, AARP Magazine, March/April 2008, Page 32, Tech Savvy

Chapter 12
KNOWING WHEN IT'S TIME FOR AN IN-HOME SITTER

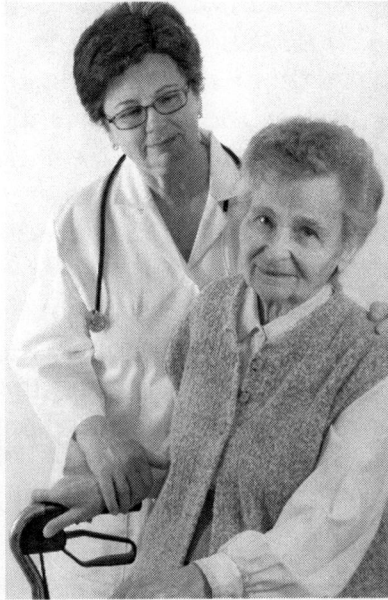

In spite of all the effort you have made to allow your loved one to maintain as normal lifestyle as possible in their home alone, there will come a time when you have only one remaining option to keep them in their home. When they are unable to perform the basic tasks of making themselves a sandwich, or pouring themselves a glass of milk, or getting dressed on their own, they will need someone to be with them to assist with these tasks. At some point they will be unable to go to the bathroom on their own recognizance or turn back their bed to go to sleep at night. They may instead, just wander about the house all night with no idea of what they are doing. They will stop eating unless coaxed to do so because they will forget how to go about the process or even where to find food. When they reach this stage, they will spend more time just sitting and staring or gazing out the window. They will spend more time sleeping at odd times and less time conversing when you try to talk to them. No longer will they think about such things, as turning on the TV or going out to get the newspaper. At this point, it's time to have someone with them most of the time. If someone, whether it be a family member, friend, someone from church, or someone else that you trust lives close by and can respond to any type of monitored emergency quickly, you could probably get by for a while longer with part-time care givers. As I mentioned before, these caregivers could be one or more members of the family, members from church, friends, but only people you trust with your life. If you have enough volunteers to cover the time periods necessary, you may be able to avoid paying for a professional caregiver at this point. Initially there probably needs to be someone there with the loved one for all three meals until they retire for the evening. This way the only time that they are alone is when they are in bed hopefully sleeping. By utilizing the electronic camera monitoring system that my sisters and I used, if they get up during the night, we could see this, and if necessary, call someone who could get there quickly. Once they begin to fail to maintain their balance and be able to walk safely, it is time to have someone stay with them 24 hours a day. The monitoring does supplement as a night person for a while, but when you are concerned with them getting up at night and falling, or falling out of bed, this is no longer an option. The task of taking care of your loved one would not be a huge task for anyone if enough people volunteered to help out. It's times like these when family and friends need to pull together for the benefit of a loved one and be able to expect the same treatment in return. Years ago there would be many more volunteers than needed, but unfortunately times have changed. Keep in mind that this doesn't have to be a permanent situation for anyone who volunteers and that you appreciate any time that anyone can devote. After you have your volunteers, you can determine how many hours or days would have to be covered by a professional caregiver. Most care giver organizations, will work with you however you would like. You can get them by the half day, day, week or even more permanent. They will also perform certain basic functions such as doing the loved one's laundry, light housekeeping, prepare them hot meals, etc. There are many caregiver organizations available but you should do a great deal of research in this area to be sure you are getting good quality care. You want to be sure that any organization you are considering is insured by your state, bonded, licensed by your state, and carries workers compensation insurance. In addition to the obvious question of how much they charge, you also want to be sure that the caregivers are actual employees of the organization and not sub-contractors. Ask some questions. Would you be under any type of contract, and if so what type and for how long? Most of these organizations simply bill you weekly and you are under no long-term contract. Be sure to ask if their caregivers' backgrounds are thoroughly checked, and that they are drug tested and experienced. Find out if they have a high turnover of employees or do they have several caregivers that have been with them for a substantial period of time. Would your loved one have the same caregiver or several different ones? Write down all the questions that are important to you before you begin to call these organizations. This way you can ask them all the same questions and have a good basis for comparison in making a decision.

Your situation may be that the finances are available to hire a full-time in-home caregiver for your loved one. In most cases, this would be the far better choice than having to place your loved one in a nursing home. If this is your situation and you are able to get good quality in home care, you are very fortunate. Keep in mind that any stranger in your loved ones home on a permanent basis will need to be at least moderately supervised by you or some member of your family from time to time. You need to constantly be aware of the day by day care they are providing. This is another reason the electronic monitoring camera system is so wonderful. You can periodically monitor what is going on in the home and feel a great degree of comfort knowing that you still have control of your loved ones life. If you don't feel the caregiver is doing the quality job you want, contact the agency for a replacement, and if you still do not feel comfortable with the person they provide, you may need to consider a different agency. Visit the Home Instead Senior Care web site at http://www.homeinstead.com/home.aspx. You can also call them at 1-888-484-5759 should you prefer. Below, I have included a list of services you can discuss in part with a potential in-home caregiver agency. There are many other services they may provide included here that should help you formulate a list for your own loved one. The first group of services would be considered Companionship Services, and these would include offering elderly companionship and conversation; provide respite care; monitor diet and eating; check food expirations; assist with evening and tuck-in; aid with morning and wake-up; arrange appointments; provide medication reminders; aid with reading; assist with walking; write letters and correspondence; organize mail;

stimulate mental awareness; assist with entertaining; answer the door; reminisce about the past; assist with clothing selection; care for houseplants; provide reminders for appointments; discuss current and historical events; participate in crafts; play games and cards; supervise home maintenance; record and arrange recipes; oversee home deliveries; prepare grocery lists; clip coupons for shopping; monitor TV usage; mail bills and letters; buy magazines, papers, and books; rent and play movies; plan visits, outings, and trips; visit neighbors and friends; read religious materials; maintain calendar; maintain family scrapbook; and record family history.

Other similar services, which could be considered Home Helper Services, would include such things as providing Alzheimer's care; assist with laundry and ironing; take out garbage; change linens; plan, prepare, and clean up meals; make beds; dust furniture; drop off and pick up dry cleaning; pick up prescriptions; organize and clean closets; assist with pet care; shop for groceries and supplies; prepare future meals; escort to appointments; accompany to lunch or dinner; escort for shopping and errands; attend plays and concerts; escort to religious services; attend club meetings and sporting events; and aid with airport tasks.

There are also, what is called Personal Services that may be required. Your loved one may need assistance with eating; grooming; dressing; bathing; incontinence; cognitive impairment; mobility; or medication reminders

Chapter 13
GOING FROM HOME TO A FACILITY IN STAGES

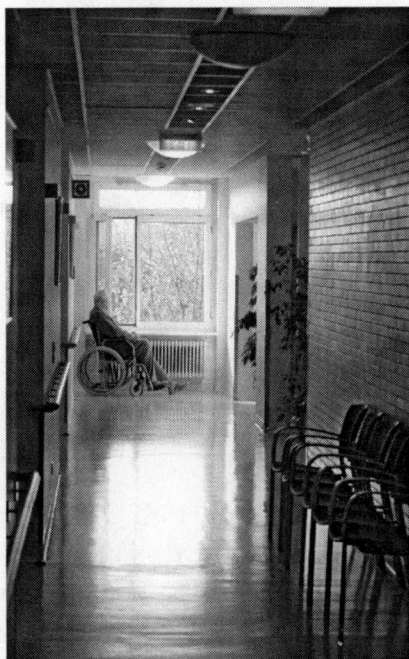

In the event that at some point your loved one does have to be moved to an assisted living facility or nursing home, don't move them straight there. Provide them with a stop off point along the way such as your own home or another member of the family's home first. Allow them a few weeks there to first get used to being out of their own home while still in the presence of those who love them. During this transition period, they will get much greater attention, care, and love while dealing with what might be a very traumatic situation for them. If they are going to be moving into a nursing home, they will surely not get the degree of initial care at a strange facility during this critical period of their life. Suddenly having to give up their home is a giant step for anyone, but no one can know exactly how your loved one in their present state of Dementia, actually feels at that point about what is happening to them. The more family and friends around them during this period the better. A good way to approach this step would be to set up a doctor's appointment for them and take them straight from their home to the doctor. Try to first explain the situation to the doctor and have him or her attempt to convince them that they need to spend the next few days with you for closer supervision and care. Let the doctor know that you would like to bring your loved one back to see him in a couple of weeks and have him explain that he wants them to go into a special care facility for a few weeks until they get stronger. If the doctor explains to them that this is what he wants them to do, they will be more reassured that it is something they need to do.

During this transition period, you should do a great deal of research into finding the best possible facility in which to place your loved one. The next stop if possible, depending on the degree of care necessary, hopefully could be an assisted living facility with an Alzheimer's unit. You can visit this web site http:// www.seniorhousingfinder.org/, and search for a facility in your area. They have over 65,000 facilities in their database. Most of these facilities allow your loved one to bring several of their own possessions such as a few pieces of furniture, TV, and other familiar items. Most of these would be private rooms with their own bathroom that would still allow them to have a little bit of home around them. Be sure to ask all of the similar questions you asked when searching for a proper caregiver. You can find a great deal of valuable information on the Alzheimer's Association's web site, located at http://www.alz.org/carefinder/index.asp to compile a list of questions to ask. In the case of an assisted living facility or a nursing home, you and other family members will want to go there and visit first to get an idea of what it is actually like. If and only if you like what you see, would you want to take further action to move your loved one into the facility. Most of these assisted living facilities are actually very nice, very well staffed, with good qualified caregivers. In the event you are able to move your loved one into an assisted living facility, in some cases it may be better not to take them to a families home first. If they go from their own home with familiar surroundings to the assisted living facility, here again with familiar items in their room, it may be less confusing for some than others. Naturally this situation would vary among different individuals and is merely food for thought. The assisted living staff will want a few days without a great deal of family intervention to earn the loved one's trust. After this initial period, try to have family and friends visit as often as possible. Co-ordinate visits with each other so no one goes at the same time if this is the only way to allow your loved one more visits. The more visitors who go at different times and spend time with them the better. At this point, the true value of family association with the loved one may not be apparent, but common sense dictates the more the merrier.

With regard to my mother's situation, we observed her fall for the last time by way of the electronic camera system and I believe that this was the straw that broke the camel's back for all three of us (my sisters and I). We all agreed that it was time to get her into a facility where she would have twenty four-hour assistance. My sister took her to the doctor who planted the seed in her mind that she needed to have closer supervision. Mother needed to hear this from a doctor or at least we felt like she did. My sister then took her home with her for a few days until she was able to take her back to the doctor for a follow up appointment. The primary purpose for this visit was for the doctor to explain to mother that he would like for her to spend a couple of weeks at a rehab type facility so she could get better. This was really just a tactic to get mother to go somewhere other than my sister's home and understand why she was going there. The doctor wanted her to do it so therefore mother was more receptive to the idea. You must understand that my sister had already explained to the doctor what we were trying to accomplish with mother so he agreed to help in this respect by encouraging her to do as we suggested. During the period when my mother was staying with my sister before this follow up doctor visit, we all discussed assisted living facilities. There was one in the town where my sister lived that she was very familiar with and even knew several of the people that worked there. We all visited the facility and talked to the staff and took a tour of the entire home. After spending some time there, we were convinced that this would be the perfect place for mother. We solidified the contract and furnished mother's room with only her own possessions. We moved in her own bed and bedroom furniture, her TV and a couple of living room items. We placed all her necessary clothes in her closet and in her dressers for when she arrived. Her room was a little larger than an average size bedroom with a large closet and bathroom. The bathroom was equipped with all the necessary orthopedic rails and shower and commode provisions, etc. We had the room smelling sweet with fresh flowers and all of her own family photos sitting around so her first impression would hopefully be a good one. The day we brought her to the room for the first time was certainly a time of much anxiety for all of us. We didn't know what to expect. We wondered if all of a sudden she would notice her own belongings and suddenly think we were trying to manipulate her life. Well the moment of truth arrived and we brought her into the room and from that moment to the day she died, she never once considered that room to be anything but a home. She may or may not have considered it her old home but we never pushed the issue. She always seemed to be content there and that made us content with our choice.

As with most assisted living facilities, they operate under certain guide lines and code restrictions. Had my mother not died of a heart attack when she did, at some point we might have had to move her into a nursing home for a more extensive level of care. If my mother's condition had worsened, and she had become unable to comply with their guide lines such as being able to vacate the building in a specified period of time in the event of a fire, she would have had to leave the facility. This is when the nursing home would have been the next step in her care. We checked into this possibility and found one that pleased us and we felt comfortable with, not far from the assisted living facility where she was living at the time. Even though she was getting excellent care at the assisted living facility, she would have received more intense medical treatment that she had begun to need, at the nursing home.

Chapter 14
HELPFUL RESOURCES

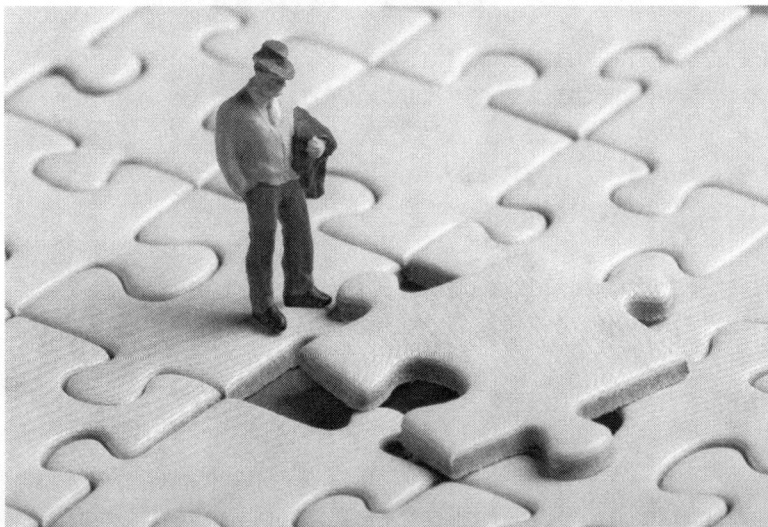

Whether you are going through the process of caring for someone with Dementia alone or with the benefit of a large support system, you should be aware of the available helpful resources. There are several different types of agencies that may be needed along the way or throughout the caregiving process. Be aware that there are adult day care facilities, in-home assistance, visiting nurses and Meals on Wheels type of organizations. You will surely learn of others by way of your association with other caregivers and people affected in some way by Dementia. Make note of these agencies and add to them as you learn of others that might help people affected by this disease. Here are a few of the more important organizations, but there are many more available. You need only do a good thorough Google search or have someone do one for you.

Alzheimer's Association 1-800-272-3900
http://www.alz.org/index.asp

Alzheimer's
http://www.pbs.org/theforgetting/symptoms/index.html

Alzheimer's Handbook
http://alzheimershandbook.com/

Alzheimer's Information Site
http://www.alzinfo.org/

The American Healthcare Foundation
http://www.alzheimers-md.org/

American Academy of Neurology
http://www.aan.com/

American Association for Geriatric Psychiatry
http://www.aagpgpa.org/

Area Agencies on Aging
http://www.n4a.org/

Assisted Living 101
http://assistedliving101.com/index.asp

Assisted Living Facilities
http://www.eldernet.com/assisted/assisted.htm

American Geriatrics Society
http://www.americangeriatrics.org/

American Medical Association
http://www.ama-assn.org/

Eldercare Locator 1-800-677-1116
http://www.eldercare.gov/Eldercare/Public/Home.asp

Consumer Consortium on Assisted Living 1-703-533-8121
http://www.ccal.org/

AARP
http://www.aarp.org/

PreventAD.com
http://www.preventad.com/

Elder Rage
http://www.elderrage.com/index.asp

U.S. Department of Veterans Affairs 1-800-827-1000
https://iris.va.gov/scripts/iris.cfg/php.exe/enduser
home.php

Financial Planning Association 1-800-322-4237
http://www.fpanet.org/public/

Family Caregiver Alliance 1-800-445-8106
http://www.caregiver.org/caregiver/jsp/home.jsp

National Academy of Elder Law Attorneys 1-520-881-4005
http://www.naela.org/

National Association of Professional Geriatric Care
Managers 1-520-881-8008
http://www.caremanager.org/

National Center on Elder Abuse 1-800-677-1116
http://www.ncea.aoa.gov/ncearoot/Main_Site/index.aspx

The Alzheimer's Store
http://www.alzstore.com/

Alzheimer's Research Forum
http://www.alzforum.org/

Alzheimer Solutions
http://alzheimersolutions.stores.yahoo.net/

Alzheimer's Directory
http://www.zarcrom.com/users/alzheimers/dirs.html

Aging Parents
http://www.agingparents.com/

Aging Parents and Elder Care
http://www.aging-parents-and-elder-care.com/

Aging Today
http://www.asaging.org/at/at-291/toc.cfm

Aging with Dignity
http://www.agingwithdignity.org/

AgingCare.com
http://www.agingcare.com/

A resource for caregivers and professionals dealing
with Alzheimer's
http://www.agelessdesign.com/

Solutions for Better Aging
http://www.agenet.com/

Agitation Test
http://www.medafile.com/zyweb/CMAI.htm

Assisted Living Locator
http://www.brookdaleliving.com/home.aspx

Assisted Living Facilities
http://www.assisted-living-directory.com/

Assisted Living Federation of America
http://www.alfa.org/i4a/pages/index.cfm?pageid=3278

At Home Care
http://www.homecareofpa.com/

Federal and state assistance programs
http://www.benefitscheckup.org/

Care Guide
http://www.careguide.com/html/home.html

Care Trak International (Monitor and locate wanderers)
http://www.caretrak.com/

Care.com (Find pre-screened caregivers in your area)
http://www.care.com/

CaregiverPros (Connects Caregivers, Employers,
Families, Clients)
http://caregiverpros.com/

Caregiving-online (Coaching, Caregiving, Live's Transitions)
http://www.caregiving-online.com/

Drugs (Catalog of FDA Approved Drug Products)
http://www.accessdata.fda.gov/scripts/cder/drugsatfda/

DyingWell.com (Defining wellness through the end of life)
http://www.dyingwell.com/

Easter Seals
http://www.easterseals.com/site/PageServer

Elderly Abuse Lawyers
http://www.elder-abuse-foundation.com/

Elder Law Answers
http://www.elderlawanswers.com/

ElderHope.com
http://www.elderhope.com/

ElderLifePlanning
http://www.elderlifeplanning.com/

ElderLink (Free Senior & Care Referral Service)
http://www.elderlink.org/index.html

Care Home Finders
http://www.carehomefinders.com/index.html

Care Pathways
http://www.carepathways.com/

To request an Instant Long Term Care Insurance Quote
http://www.long-term-care-quote.com/quote.html

To request a Life Insurance Quote
http://www.life-insurance-coverage.com/quote.html

A Place for Mom (search for eldercare)
http://www.aplaceformom.com/assess.asp?SID=54

Senior Health Guide
http://seniorhealth.about.com/library/weekly/aa101401a.htm

Accent on Seniors
http://www.accentonseniors.com/

Benefits Checkup
http://www.benefitscheckup.org/

Legal Assistance available by state
http://www.abanet.org/aging/resources/statemap.shtml

Licensing Agencies by state
http://www.nursinghomeaction.com/static_pages/help.cfm

Access to Benefits Coalition
http://www.accesstobenefits.org/

Exercise equipment for the disabled
http://www.accesstr.com/

Alternative Solutions in Long Term Care
http://www.activitytherapy.com/

Medicare and You 1-800-633-4227
http://www.medicare.gov/Publications/Pubs/pdf/10050.pdf

National Long Term Care Ombudsman 1-202-332-2275
http://www.ltcombudsman.org/static_pages/ombudsmen.cfm

Nursing Home Compare
http://www.cms.hhs.gov/CertificationandComplianc/12_NHs.asp

Personal Health Record 1-312-233-1100
http://www.myphr.com/

SNAP for Seniors 1-800-651-7627
http://www.snapforseniors.com/

CARING TODAY 1-203-254-0783
http://www.caringtoday.com/

Home Instead Senior Care 1-888-484-5759
http://www.homeinstead.com/home.aspx

National Family Caregivers Association 1-800-896-3650
www.thefamilycaregiver.org

ADT Companion Service 1-800-209-7599
www.adt.com or www.aarp.org/adtcompanion

Family Caregiver Alliance/National Center on Caregiving
1-800-445-8106
www.caregiver.org

The Alzheimer's Foundation of America
http://www.alzfdn.org/

National Institute on Aging
http://www.nia.nih.gov/alzheimers

National Alzheimer's Association 1-800-272-3900
www.alz.org

Administration on Aging 1-202-619-0724
www.aoa.dhhs.gov

Chapter 15
KNOW IN YOUR HEART,
YOU DID YOUR BEST

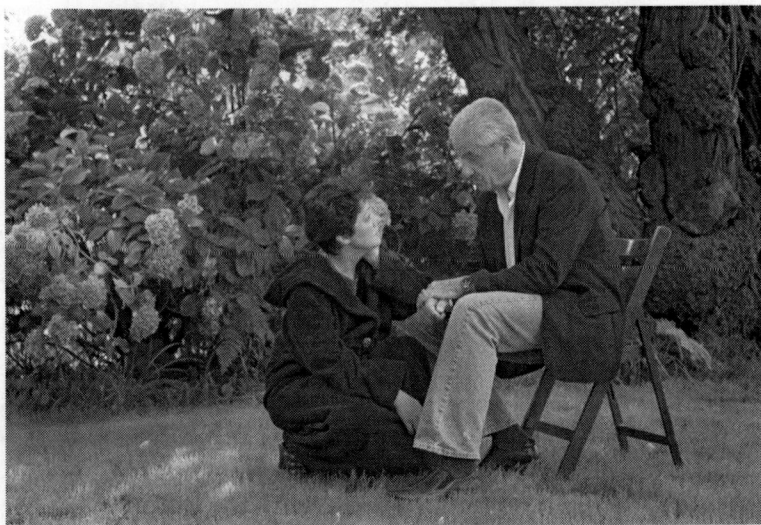

At some point there will possibly come a time when you begin to feel that their condition is totally out of your hands and that your efforts no longer make a difference. Don't allow this feeling to take control of you. Hold on to the fact that as long as there is breath in their body, you can affect their life, if only in some small way. Continue to spend time with them, continue to talk to them, and continue to assist them in any way you can. You may not realize you are making any vital contributions or doing them any good, but keep in mind that they may realize more than you know. You may not think they hear what you say or know who you are, but you don't really know this to be true. Even though there comes a time when they cease to speak to you or seem to merely stare out the window at nothing, in their heart they may hold you dear to them. They may mentally be in another world, but for all we know they may have us there with them. When my mother passed away, one of my sister's held one of her hands, I held the other and my other sister was stroking her hair as she took her last breath. We all feel a great deal of comfort knowing that there is nothing we know of that we either failed to do for her or didn't at least try to do for her that needed to be done during her illness. During my mother's illness, her needs were foremost in our minds at all times. We were constantly asking ourselves; What does she need? or Would this be better for her than something else? When should we implement this into her care? How much longer will it be until she will have to have this? Its' also very comforting to know that because of our collective efforts, our mother was able to enjoy a good deal more life than she otherwise would have been able to. There is still so much we don't know about Dementia/Alzheimers. Because of this, we are still allowed the luxury of believing what we wish to believe about certain aspects of it. By spending all the quality time you can with them, you will know in your heart that you did everything you possibly could for them while they were in your life. This is and always has been extremely important to my family and me. We loved our mother dearly and we showed her right up to the very end of her life.

"YOU MAY NOT REMEMBER ME,
BUT I WILL ALWAYS REMEMBER YOU."

A Little About the Author

In order to tell you a little about myself, I must first explain who I am not. I have no medical credentials, nor am I a world famous author. To put it another way, I am no one special, but merely one of millions of people who have been affected in some way by the diseases known as Alzheimer's. In my case, I, along with my two sisters, spent the last six years providing care to our now deceased 86-year-old mother who had the disease. She was a wonderful woman, whom my sisters and I watched go from the initial stages to the advanced stages in this brief period of time. Over the past six years, I have learned a great deal about Dementia and how best to care for someone who has it. I learned quickly that one of the most important goals would be to figure out ways to keep our mother in her own home as long as safely possible. I had a good support system through this entire process that is so very important. Having been raised in a Christian home in a small community called Only, Tennessee, we have always been a close family. Although we lost our father in 1974, our mother had always remained our foundation. I'm 62 years old and grew up during the 50's and 60's, when family values were quite different from what they are now. Not only was our immediate family close, but our extended family and friends as well. If anyone in the family got sick or hurt, everyone including our friends were concerned about helping out. Most of us "Baby Boomers", as we are commonly referred to, still feel this way. When you are fortunate enough to have other family members all helping to achieve the common goal as I have, it is less stressful on everyone. This allowed us to individually focus on more positive aspects of our mother's care. It also allowed us to figure out ways to more easily deal with each problem that arose with mother's disease. The things we learned along the way became the reason for this book. One thing I learned was how many people were going through the same things we were, but in many cases with very little of the knowledge we had acquired. I have simply tried to pour my heart out to anyone who feels the need for the information I have chosen to share.

Bibliography

Photo Sources
Melanie Townsend Graphic Artist / Layout & Design

Information Sources
Mary Townsend
Canita Campbell
Cindy Parker
Linda Townsend
Sue Anne Stutts
Mary Carolyn McClanahan
Wallace & Judy Embry

Jacqueline Marcell
http://www.elderrage.com/index.asp

Alzheimer's Association http://www.alz.org/index.asp
24/7 Helpline
Contact us for information, referral and support.
tel: 1-800-272-3900
tdd: 1-866-403-3073
e-mail: info@alz.org

Dr. Russell Blaylock, a Physician, Neurosurgeon,
Author, Lecturer, and Health Advocate
http://www.russellblaylockmd.com/

James Joseph, director of the neuroscience lab at the
USDA Human Nutrition Research Center on Aging at
Tufts University

US News and World Report www.usnews.com

Caring Today www.caringtoday.com

Waneen Spirduso, Ed.D., professor at the University of Texas at Austin, and author of Exercise and Its Mediating Effects on Cognition (Human Kinetics, 2007).

AARP www.aarp.com

The AARP Magazine http://www.aarpmagazine.org/

Researchers at the University of Illinois

Researchers at Columbia University

Home Instead Senior Care 1-888-484-5759
http://www.homeinstead.com/home.aspx

Telecommunications Devices Access Program or T.D.A.P. TDAP.TRA@STATE.TN.US

Tennessee Regulatory Agency, 460 James Robertson Parkway, Nashville, Tennessee 37243-0505

ADT Security Services, Inc
http://www.adt.com/wps/portal/adt/global/

Technical Sources
Melanie Townsend—Graphic Artist / Layout & Design
Linda Townsend—Editor

CPSIA information can be obtained at www.ICGtesting.com
Printed in the USA
LVOW071408220911

247388LV00002B/296/P

9 781606 722565